Proverbs 31 Prepper

Proverbs 31 Prepper

by Annette Reeder
The Biblical Nutritionist™

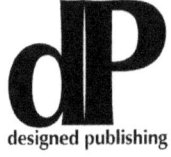

©2015, 2022 by Annette Reeder. All rights reserved.
Designed Publishing, a division of
Designed Healthy Living,
Glen Allen, Virginia, 23059

No part of this publication may be reproduced, stored in a retrieval system, or transmitted in any way by any means—electronic, mechanical, photocopy, recording, or otherwise—without the prior permission of the copyright holder, except as provided by USA copyright law.

Unless otherwise noted, all Scriptures are taken from the
New American Standard Bible,
© 1960, 1963, 1968, 1971, 1972, 1973, 1975, 1977, 2022
by the Lockman Foundations.
Used by permission.

ISBN: 978-1-7376278-1-4

Library of Congress Control Number: 2017907965

Disclaimer:
Being a nutritionist I must state that the medical statements in this book, specifically the medical herbal recommendations, do not offer medical advice or replace medical attention. This book has not been approved or read by the FDA or any other government agency.

Proverbs 31:10-31

An excellent wife, who can find?

For her worth is far above jewels.

The heart of her husband trusts in her,
and he will have no lack of gain.

She does him good and not evil all the days of her life.

She looks for wool and flax, and works with her hands in delight.

She is like merchant ships; she brings her food from afar.

She rises also while it is still night, and gives food
to her household, and portions to her maidens.

She considers a field and buys it; from her
earnings she plants a vineyard.

She girds herself with strength, and makes her arms strong.

She senses that her gain is good; her lamp does not go out at night.

She stretches out her hands to the distaff,
and her hands grasp the spindle.

She extends her hand to the poor; and
she stretches out her hands to the needy.

She is not afraid of the snow for her household,
for all her household are clothed with scarlet.

She makes coverings for herself;
her clothing is fine linen and purple.

Strength and dignity are her clothing
and she smiles at the future.

She opens her mouth in wisdom and
the teaching of kindness is on her tongue.

She looks well to the ways of her household
and does not eat the bread of idleness.

Her children rise up and bless her;
her husband also, as he praises her saying,
"Many daughters have done nobly, but you excel them all."

Charm is deceitful and beauty is vain,
but a woman who fears the Lord shall be praised.

Give her the product of her hands,
and let her works praise her in the gates.

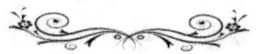

Table of Contents

Introduction 3

Part A
Getting Started 9

    Pray 9

    Plan 9

    Put Into Action 10

    Practice. 10

    Who is Jesus to You? 12

Menu Planning 15

    One Week Menu. 18

    One Month Menu Divided into 4 Weeks 24

    Six Months – One Year. 28

    Inventory. 31

    Inventory Notes 34

    Meal Necessities 35

    Pray 35

    72 Hours. 38

- Cooking 41
  - Short Term Options 41
  - Long Term Options 44
  - Kitchen Supplies 47
  - Appliances 48
- Gardening 51
  - Raised Bed Gardening – aka Square Foot Gardening 52
  - Wood Chip Gardening 53
  - Container Gardening 53
  - Indoor Gardening 55
- Preserving Food 61
  - Water-Bath Canning 62
  - Steam Pressure Canning 63
  - Freezing 64
  - Adjustments for High-Altitude Canning 65
  - Tips for Successful and Safe Canning 66
  - Dehydrating 66
  - Freeze Dried 68
- Recipes 71
- Cleaning 77
  - DIY Homemade Cleaners 78
  - Now for the Easy - Organic – Simple Solution 81
- Medicine/Herbal Medicine Cabinet 85
  - First Aid Kits 86

Table of Contents

    Building an Herbal Medicine Cabinet 86

Dan Celia Comments 89

Praising 95

Worshipping 103

    I Spied God Today 103

    An Amen Day 104

    Bible Verses 105

Partnering 107

Part B

    Dehydration Tips 109

    LeQuip Filter Pro Dehydrator 112

    Benefits of Apple Cider Vinegar 114

    Epsom Salt Uses 118

    Baking Soda Uses 121

    Hydrogen Peroxide 124

    Top 64 Uses of a Bandana for Survival and Prepping 127

    Canning Recipes 130

Resources 133

Notes 135

About the Author 145

Other Books by Annette Reeder 147

Introduction

The Proverbs 31 woman is one of strong character, great wisdom, many skills and deep compassion. She is one who is prepared *and* praised.

Today we **can be** that woman. Today we **need to be** that woman.

Our world is full of unrest. Because of this unrest we need to take another look at the verses in Proverbs 31. Each verse teaches strength of character in being prepared.

She **brings** her food from afar

She **makes** coverings for herself

She **looks well** to the ways of her household

She **girds** herself with strength

She is **not afraid** of the snow for her household

The Proverbs 31 woman was prepared.

Years ago I thought I was a prepared mother if I remembered the sunscreen for our trip to the beach and if I had the school supplies ready *before* school started.

Priorities in Preparing

It seems like the first 50 years of my life has passed in a blur, what seemed important at the time has been replaced with other seemingly important matters. An accumulation of my life's lessons came down to two priorities beyond my own personal salvation: have I prepared my family and have I reached out to those around me?

I am not striving to be praised in the gates as it says in Proverbs 31; instead I am striving to be faithfully prepared. And how do we find ourselves faithfully prepared with the unrest in America and around the world?

We can be found faithful as we accept that God has placed us here at this time for this reason. His plan is unfolding before us. We could have been born in the 1800's. Think of the problems and blessings they encountered back then. But no, God chose for us to be alive – truly alive – at such a time as this. It is His design we are here today.

And since this is our time and our place, we are to live it fully and keep on preparing.

We must work the works of Him who sent Me as long as it is day; night is coming when no man can work. John 9:4

How does a family prepare?

Today in troubled times the coined word for preparing is prepper. Prepper is defined as a person who believes a catastrophic disaster or emergency is likely to occur in the future and makes active preparations for it.

I do not totally agree with how some authors and websites use the term prepper; to go off grid, hide in a cave, store enough food and ammunition for an army. Instead a Proverbs 31 Prepper is one who has prepared her family well and will not face storms without common sense and supplies.

How do we as the caretakers of our homes make sure our family is ready for the snow? How do we care for one of the most important provisions – food — without negating the basic need of quality nutrition? How do we become the Proverbs 31 Prepper, someone who is ready for emergencies?

Simple, we step back in time and envision the life of our grandmothers. My grandmother once canned over 1200 jars in one summer. I cannot imagine that happening in my kitchen since the whistle and steam of the pressure canner still scares me. Thankfully she had 10 children over the years which provided a perfect team of helpers.

{ *She is not afraid of the snow for her household, for all her household are clothed with scarlet.* }

Today I can still visit that century old farm house and carefully go

Introduction

down those rough wooden steps into the cellar. "Watch your head" my grandmother would always say. And if I use my memory well I can see those canned jars filled with every vegetable and fruit imaginable on the stacked wooden shelves. The peaches, apples, corn, green beans, just name it, and it was there. My grandmother was prepared. She worked hard and she did her work with grace and without complaining.

Although my grandmother prepared, it was preparation for 'normal life'. Feed the family well and they prosper. Today we need to prepare families to prosper although this task may not seem so *normal*.

There are two basic reasons to be prepared

The first is to **better feed our families nutrient dense foods.** As I teach across the country in churches, I share the message of our biggest mistake as Christian mothers: giving up control of our most precious commodity – food – to the government and manufacturers. We stopped listening and learning from grandmother and started absent mindedly obeying the men in the white lab coats. The more processed foods became accepted the more disease processes we acquired. We are plagued with diseases today that were unheard of 50 years ago. We are not winning the battle against cancer; we are funding it with the purchase of processed foods. Our children are more harmed by poor diet today than drugs, alcohol and tobacco combined. While we would not give a baby a beer we do give them drug altered foods that are just as toxic.

To prepare for difficult times many 'prepper' sites suggest buying food that is far from superior in quality. Instead it is about cheap food that will leave your family stressed and malnourished. As I am going to teach you, whether this food becomes your normal daily nourishment rotated throughout the year or stored for storms, it needs to be a quality that your family will be healthy consuming. During difficult times is not when you want stomach issues or headaches which are typical with processed foods.

Secondly, having **food on hand brings confidence** when the storms come. And storms are coming – fast. Storms can be in the tumultuous weather, the impending collapse of the economy or the quickly eroding morality.

It wasn't until I got married that I learned to run to the grocery store when a storm was coming. My mother was always well stocked with groceries. When the snows came she pulled out some of our favorite foods. As a foodie from birth I looked forward to storms. I can even remember cooking on the wood stove in our basement and eating by candle light during a snow storm power outage. It wasn't romantic but it was fun.

When a family is prepared, like my mom was, storms are not chaotic. My mom was a Proverbs 31 woman.

Weather

Today it is typical to get a 3 day warning when snow storms or hurricanes are heading our way. That means race to the store and stock up on the essentials such as bread, milk, cereal, and toilet paper, and also the non-essentials such as videos, chips, cookies, and candy. What if you lived in Oklahoma when the tornado came through and caused disaster? Or Joplin, Missouri where the tornado cleared a one mile stretch of homes and businesses? No warning, no stocking up, and no food to feed your family.

> *But understand this that in the last days there will come times of difficulty. 2 Timothy 3:1*

Economy

In the 80's my husband and I were both being threatened with job loss. We were newly married in our first small 4 room home with an 18% mortgage interest rate. With our jobs threatened we decided to not use any appliances or unnecessarily spend money. It was one of the hottest summers on record in St. Louis. So instead of using the air conditioner we sat in the back yard on those blue plastic tri-fold lawn chairs with our feet up and with the water sprinkler swinging back and forth, keeping us cool with its water. Our neighbors thought we were the newlyweird newlyweds. Our meals were peanut butter sandwiches – almost every day. When the layoff happened I was 2 people above the lay off line and Steve found a new job before his current job closed the doors.

As it turned out we didn't miss any paychecks but yet we had no way of knowing what the outcome would be. The same is true today, trials will come but how each one of us will be affected is not known.

In the summer of 2015 Greece was seeing an economic meltdown. Each citizen could get in a line for hours to withdraw only $66. Can you imagine living on $66 a day? What food would you buy? What bills would you pay? Stores are closed – what would you eat? Businesses are closed - how would you earn money? Can this economic disaster happen in America? Many predict it could happen overnight.

In America our own government is pleasing the few at the expense of the many. Our healthcare is determined by bureaucrats not our physicians. The Judeo Christian foundation that made America abundant and strong is crumbling. Our Constitution which was based on God's laws is being used as wall paper. We are being ruled by man and not laws. All while the good are being called evil and the evil are being praised. (Isaiah 5:20)

> *Knowing this first of all, that scoffers will come in the last days with scoffing, following their own sinful desires.*
> *2 Peter 3:3*

Even our dollar is being artificially manipulated to appear strong while being propped up with fake reports. All it will take for America to become an economic ruin is for the prop to be removed. The dominoes will fall.

Political/Principles

The nerves of many people in our country are frayed. Violence erupts with little notice. The George Floyd event was evidence of this. Without hesitation people took to the streets and rioted for causes most did not even understand. People are unsettled. Yet these riots are not the answer. They bring no justice and since the riots, chaos continues and crime has multiplied.

On June 26, 2015, our country saw the beginning of judiciary abuse. A panel of 9 judges decided to vote for the minority to judge the majority with the first ever ruling on the land that mandates gays as equal in marriage. And yet the ink is still wet and the line is forming for polygamy and pedophiles claiming their equal justice. The very fabric of our country is not gradually unraveling; it is being torn to shreds.

In the same summer as the marriage disorder we saw on national TV how babies alive and dead are being dismembered and sold to the highest bidder.

Envy, drunkenness, orgies, and things like these.
I warn you, as I warned you before, that those who do
such things will not inherit the kingdom of God. Galatians 5:21

Alarms have been sounding. America must turn back to God. The weather is brewing, the terrorists are engaging, and Scripture is warning. America must turn back to God.

Many highly respected financial analysts are predicting an economic Armageddon. America must turn back to God.

I must stay tuned to God. I must prepare my family for troubled times ahead. I must prepare so I can share the Gospel with those who are not prepared physically or spiritually.

Watch therefore, and pray always that you may be counted
worthy to escape all these things that will come to pass, and
to stand before the Son of Man. Luke 21:36 (NKJV)

Today

We know the final act of this story but we don't know when our role is complete. Will the economic disaster that has been predicted for years actually happen? Will we be raptured before the chaos sets in? Will life continue as is for another 20 years? Good questions. I don't have the answers. I know being prepared means I don't need to fret about 'what-ifs' when the 'therefores' will get me through.

But the end of all things is at hand:
be ye therefore sober, and watch unto prayer. 1 Peter 4:7

Be patient therefore, brethren, unto the coming of the Lord.
Behold, the husbandman waiteth for the precious fruit of the earth, and hath
long patience for it, until he receive the early and latter rain. James 5:7

Introduction

The confidence of being prepared brings peace of mind and ability to serve.

Remember my concern is to make sure my family is ready for the future – both spiritually and physically. And then I am to be eager and commanded to reach out to others.

What about you, why do you want to be prepared?

*She is like merchant ships; she **brings** her food from afar. Proverbs 31:14*

This book will cover the **4 necessary steps to implement**: pray, plan, put into action and practice. These steps are simple, practical and essential. So grab your favorite apron and put on comfortable shoes, because the kitchen is going to be your new entertainment room. Be sure and invite others to join in.

We are traveling back to the future. Memories are about to be made. Blessings are waiting to happen.

The Proverbs 31 woman was prepared.

So let's start prepping!

Getting Started

Pray

From gardening to cooking, from preparing to saving; each of these topics come with suggestions, options, and how-to's. Read each section of this workbook and pray about the options and implementation. Learning new cooking and preparing options may be overwhelming. God will guide you. From there the planning will be simple.

{ Strength and dignity are her clothing and she **smiles** at the future. }

Plan

How many times do I find myself in the grocery store without a plan only to fill my cart with instant, ready to eat foods or vegetables that look great and inviting only to rot in my refrigerator because I don't have a plan for their use? Yes, when I shop without a plan I make more trips throughout the week and have more food wasted than my budget allows.

So how do we plan not only for a week, or a month or even a year? How do we plan for unknown future happenings? Easy – we go back in time and forget our convenient and "just in time" mentality. Think like our grandmother. What is in season, what is on sale that is nutritious and what does my family like? The chapters in this workbook will be a guide to write a list, inventory supplies and then prepare a plan. From there we are prepared to prepare.

No one goes to the grocery store the day after a snow fall expecting to fill their list. Instead it pays to plan ahead, have food ready and store the provisions in a handy place. Planning prevents chaos.

{ Planning prevents chaos. }

Each section in this workbook will give ideas for plans to prosper.

Put Into Action

I am notorious for making plans, write them out on sticky notes only to let them slip off my goal board and disappear under my desk. Therefore "out of sight out of mind". To be prepared we must put into action the plans. Plans without action fail. Each chapter in this workbook will include simple action steps. This is very important.

Practice

We teach our children how to escape the home if a fire happens. We teach our children when they are young to dial 911. These are important safety measures so we practice them, again and again. The same is true for preparing for emergencies, cooking without power, feeding our family without the convenience of our favorite appliances. We need to practice. Practice brings peace of mind.

This book will give insight into options for cooking, gardening and preserving. Choose the ones most likely to succeed in your kitchen and then practice to perfect it. Perfect it not only for the delivery of delicious taste but for the ease of preparing.

Choose a meal each week to practice prepping skills. Then choose one day a month to practice all meals. Invite the family to join in the fun by using paper plates, eating with candles, and telling stories instead of watching TV.

Now is the time to practice gardening skills and preserving techniques. Surprises wait as fun and adventure are about to happen.

Pray

I started with prayer and I am repeating it here with a different emphasis.

There are times in our life that bring more challenges than others. As an expectant parent it was a challenge to not think about the what-ifs of being a parent. In my marriage there are what-ifs. In our careers there are what-ifs. Life is filled with what-ifs.

The topic of prepping brings new 'what-ifs' and a new level of anxiousness. What may happen for me to need this knowledge? The 'what-ifs' can be paralyzing.

Be anxious for nothing, but in everything by prayer and supplication with thanksgiving let your requests be made known to God. And the peace of God, which surpasses all comprehension, will guard your hearts and your minds in Christ Jesus. Philippians 4:6-7

Prayer starts with you. How is your relationship with the Lord? Do you *really* know who Jesus is to *You*? It is by knowing Him that brings peace. This peace will then transfer to the entire family. So again, let me ask "Who is Jesus to You?"

Who is Jesus to You?

Is He someone you sing about *or* sing to?

Is He someone you talk about *or* talk to?

Is He someone who loves others *or* loves you?

Is He someone who lives *or* lives in you?

Is He someone you visit on Sunday *or*
take with you every day?

Is He someone who died for others *or* died for you?

Jesus is…

The One who knew you before your parents.

The One who designed your blonde hair and freckles.

The One who gave you those dimples.

The One who held your hand the first day of school.

The One who stopped that car from hitting you.

The One who nudged your heart to
not fall for the devil's schemes.

The One who allowed you to cry
when someone wronged you.

The One who helps you smile and know everything will be ok when the
doctor gives you bad news.

The One who walks beside you in court.

The One who carries you during the
funeral of your mother.

The One who pays the bills when
the funds seem too short.

The One who placed the clouds in the sky
to shelter you and be beautiful.

The One who causes the rain to bring life into plants.

Introduction

The One who walked on the dry dusty roads bringing the message of salvation to everyone who would hear.

The One who sat on the Moses seat in the temple and taught the Words of the Father.

The One who caused the Red Sea to part so His children can pass on dry land.

The One who heals.

The One who listens.

The One who taught us true love.

The One who fed the 5,000.

The One who taught us blessings.

The One who calms waters.

The One who will not allow evil to flourish.

The One who will right wrongs.

The One that teaches.

The One who cries.

The One who dances.

The One who intercedes.

The One who walked up stone steps carrying a large rough timber on his raw open torn flesh and let men drive nails into his hands and feet.

The One who shared the Gospel to the dying man beside him on the cross.

The One who is coming back for us to take us home.

The One who loves us most.

He is Jesus.

Pray for family members and their relationship with the Lord. Do they know Jesus?

Pray for those around you – neighbors, coworkers, and friends. Do they know Jesus?

Pray for God to bring a passion into your soul that allows no sleep until you have reached out to people with the Gospel.

> Rejoice always; **pray without ceasing**; in everything give thanks; for this is God's will for you in Christ Jesus. I Thessalonians 5:16 - 18

The last chapter in this book is Praising. Please don't overlook this chapter. During times of stress Praise to the Lord is necessary. Included are words to popular Christian songs, Bible verses and a place to journal what God is doing.

> But He answered them, "My Father is working until now, and I Myself am working." John 5:17

God is at work at all times. Pray expectantly. Pray obediently.

Menu Planning

"What's for dinner?" What goes through your mind when you hear those words? They are at the top of the list - along with "Are we there yet?"- as the expected and yet annoying questions.

Plan

Friday night at our home is typically "pizza night." So when Steve comes home from work his first words after my kiss are typically "What's for dinner?" with the hopes for our traditional homemade pizza.

{ She looks for wool and flax, and works with her hands in delight. }

What are family favorites or food traditions?

Now is a good time to list family favorite foods, spices and traditions. Include these as much as possible during difficult times.

List family favorites:

Do some members of the family have a favorite that would 'make their day'? List them here:

What spices are used on a regular basis?

What spices are used randomly?

Planning to feed the family through a short storm or a long economic drought starts with likes and variety.

In real estate they say there are three things that matter: location, location, location. In food prepping there are three things that matter: variety, variety, variety.

I shared the story of Steve and me eating peanut butter sandwiches for months with an expected lay off approaching. Well, I must say, I was done with peanut butter. To prevent a mono diet let's prepare a menu and then stock a pantry of foods that will delight plus nourish - maybe not in that order.

Now that we know favorites, let's move on to the menu.

Write out a menu for one week. Include variety but also be smart with cooking options. Aim for simple to prepare and edible for no waste. Also, keep in mind that power may be off so do not include convenience in preparation or refrigerator items.

Menu Planning

Here is mine as an example:

Day	Breakfast	Lunch	Dinner
Sunday	Granola with powdered milk, dried blueberries	Peanut butter sandwich, dried apple slices	Popcorn
Monday	Oatmeal, raisins, nuts	Tuna salad sandwich, carrots (rehydrated), fruit	Cheddar shells with added dried ground beef and dried vegetables, applesauce
Tuesday	Cereal with powdered milk, fruit	Soup, fruit	Spaghetti, applesauce, pickles
Wednesday	Protein smoothie	Sunflower seed butter and banana sandwich	Chili
Thursday	Eggs	Hummus, vegetables on tortillas	Tortilla casserole – baked on grill.
Friday	Oatmeal, dried fruit, protein powder	Bean salad with added rehydrated vegetables	Pizza
Saturday	Granola with dried fruit	Salmon Patties, vegetables and fruit	Sloppy joes, bread, green beans, applesauce

One Week Menu

Write your 7 day menu here (use pencil)

	Breakfast	Lunch	Dinner
Sunday			
Monday			
Tuesday			
Wednesday			

Menu Planning

	Breakfast	Lunch	Dinner
Thursday			
Friday			
Saturday			

To add variety and plan beyond one week write out ten different breakfast options. I usually drink the same protein smoothie every day. But situations may arise when the smoothie is not an option so planning other food options will make me better prepared.

Write out a list of 10 different breakfasts: (use pencil)

1.

2.

3.

4.

5.

6.

7.

8.

9.

10.

Menu Planning

The same as breakfast make a list of ten options for lunches and dinners.

Write out a list of 10 lunch options: (use pencil)

1.

2.

3.

4.

5.

6.

7.

8.

9.

10.

Write out a list of 10 dinner options: (use pencil)

1.

2.

3.

4.

5.

6.

7.

8.

9.

10.

List favorite beverages. List in order of importance or nutritional value.

1.

2.

3.

4.

5.

I encourage using a pencil throughout this workbook in order to make changes as new material is learned about which foods store well and what foods to avoid. Keep adjusting the list as new discoveries are found. Sales at the store will also lend to adjusting the list as well. It doesn't matter if a meal is a family favorite if the ingredients don't store well.

Foods that are packaged in cans, foil containers, or that are home canned have a long shelf life. Foods prepared in boxes, frozen or refrigerated have a shorter shelf life.

Now, taking the menu ideas from the list of 10 makes it easy to write out a one month plan.

One Month Menu Divided into 4 Weeks

Week 1	Breakfast	Lunch	Dinner	Snacks
Sunday *Beverages*				
Monday *Beverages*				
Tuesday *Beverages*				
Wednesday *Beverages*				
Thursday *Beverages*				
Friday *Beverages*				
Saturday *Beverages*				

Menu Planning

Week 2	Breakfast	Lunch	Dinner	Snacks
Sunday *Beverages*				
Monday *Beverages*				
Tuesday *Beverages*				
Wednesday *Beverages*				
Thursday *Beverages*				
Friday *Beverages*				
Saturday *Beverages*				

Week 3	Breakfast	Lunch	Dinner	Snacks
Sunday *Beverages*				
Monday *Beverages*				
Tuesday *Beverages*				
Wednesday *Beverages*				
Thursday *Beverages*				
Friday *Beverages*				
Saturday *Beverages*				

Menu Planning

Week 4	Breakfast	Lunch	Dinner	Snacks
Sunday *Beverages*				
Monday *Beverages*				
Tuesday *Beverages*				
Wednesday *Beverages*				
Thursday *Beverages*				
Friday *Beverages*				
Saturday *Beverages*				

Six Months – One Year

Here is a list of suggested staples to have on hand:

Food per person	1 month	6 months	1 year
Beans	16 pounds	96 pounds	200 pounds
Grains	16 pounds	96 pounds	200 pounds
Fruits	25 pounds	150 pounds	300 pounds
Veggies	25 pounds	150 pounds	150 pounds
Meat	12 pounds	72 pounds	144 pounds
Salt	½ pound	2.5 pounds	5 pounds
Oil	2.5 pounds	15 pounds	30 pounds
Water	31 gallons	187 gallons	375 gallons

Keep in mind that grains includes all grains: rice, pasta, wheat, spelt, oats, etc.

This does not include spices, herbs or other flavorings.

Putting It Into Action: Write out the menu for one week, and then continue to add on more days and weeks till a full month is completed. It is easier to do inventory when the menu is completed. It will show what is needed to make that meal happen. While doing the inventory make notes of which meals are possible now and which ones need more ingredients.

After the one month plan is completed check off each day when the ingredients are prepared and ready.

Menu Planning

Here is an example of two days completed and checked.

Friday Beverages Water tea	√ Tuna salad, bread √ Carrots dehydrated Apple slices Sprouts on the tuna salad
Saturday Beverages Water Apple juice	Taco soup √ Crackers Add dried vegetables to soup √ Pudding

Inventory

The very first step in building a pantry for long term provisions is to do inventory of what is on hand.

Pull out everything from cabinets and closets. Remember how you kept putting off cleaning out the pantry? Well, today is the day to make that happen. Record each item while checking expiration dates. Put items with the shortest shelf life at the front to be used first.

If there are items not categorized here then add them to the blank pages that follow.

Baking supplies	On Hand	Need to Supply
Baking powder		
Baking soda		
Salt		
Yeast		
Dry Goods		
Pasta		
Rice		
Beans		
Black beans		
Pinto beans		

Garbanzo beans

White navy beans

_____

_____

_____

Meat – dried, canned and frozen

                                                                    On Hand   Need

Protein – powder, granola

Vegetables
Canned, dried, etc. List here.

Fruits
Canned, dried, etc. List here.

Treats – cookies, chips, etc.

Jars of sauce – pesto, marinara, salsa, etc.

Inventory

                                                          On Hand   **Need**

Mixes

Grains

Spices

Everything else

Inventory Notes

Meal Necessities

Meals need to include the three major food groups: Protein, Fats and Carbohydrates - in that order.

Protein – make sure each meal has protein as its main course. Protein is the building block for every cell in the body. Growth and immunity require protein.

Protein options include: beans, legumes, grains, meat, dairy, cheese, nuts, seeds, and nut butters.

Fats are essential! Without fats the body cannot synthesize the proper level of hormones. Hormones are the communication between cells and organs. Healthful fats contribute to soft skin, mental clarity, happiness, hair and nails soft and not brittle. When fats are missing other symptoms include heart and digestive issues.

Fats to add to the menu include: nuts, seeds, olive oil, coconut oil and other organic oils.

Carbohydrates are easy to have on hand and they help supply energy and satiety. Beans, grains, crackers, rice, vegetables and many other foods will keep us satisfied during times of difficulty.

Pray

As I was doing this activity for my own family I realized my budget was going to be stretched. Even when I teach healthy living in the churches someone will always raise the concern that eating healthy is too expensive. Here is how God has supplied my needs.

I was working on my list of foods to store and realized that milk was not fully stocked. The reason was quality milk is hard to acquire. Powdered milks are usually American dairy milk that is ultra-pasteurized. I prefer two options: raw milk and grain milks.

Raw milk is only legal in Virginia if I own a cow. Steve has made it clear

— we are not getting a cow! So my next option is milk made from grains or nuts such as Almond Milk, Oat Milk, etc. These can be expensive when stocking up. God knew my heart and He heard my prayer. The week I prayed about this asking God to show me a plan for milk, the grain milks were on clearance in the grocery store. I paid $.77 for each carton! Normally they are $2.49. The expiration dates were in February, March and June of next year. The manager said these milks were not well received so they were discontinuing them. That was a blessing. God will supply all our needs according to His riches in glory — or Kroger!

He has done this with almost every item I need to stock. Don't think for a moment that He doesn't care about your well-being. He does.

He wants to give you the desires of your heart when we pray for our life to match His will.

How to store? Let me just briefly share quick tips on storage.

The basic 5 ways:

1 – Packing in pails with oxygen absorbers

2 – Purchasing canned foods

3 – Purchasing #10 freeze-dried cans

4 – Canning (covered later in this book)

5 – Dehydrating (covered later in this book)

Packing in Pails

Certain foods are great for packing in plastic, food-grade pails (or buckets). These can be purchased or possibly obtained free at a local grocery store or bakery.

Gamma lids make getting into the buckets easier than the regular lids. Plus the Gamma lids will last a lifetime on buckets. (Can be bought at www.uline.com)

Foods that store well in buckets are grains and beans. Lentils and oats store successfully as well. Oxygen absorbers are needed to help keep the food fresh long term, and you will need Mylar (or metalized) bags. These are extra-strong bags that keep all air out long term. (www.uline.com)

Canned Foods

Many canned foods are good for at least a year. Canned meats, specifically salmon, frequently have dates out 4-5 years from the date of purchase. If canned foods are on the menu regularly, it is a good plan to have extra on hand.

Canned foods such as beans are good for the 72 hour emergency food.

#10 Freeze Dried Cans

Some freeze dried foods are pretty economical, especially on sale. The shelf life is 25 years. Freeze dried meats are also a very prudent purchase.

We cover canning and dehydrating in the chapters in this book.

Other foods to store:
- Canned fruit
- Boxed Mac & cheese
- Sauces – pasta, pesto and salsa
- Small size condiments

Put Into Action – 72 Hour Bag

Our first action step after doing inventory is to prepare for a 72 hour emergency. Most preppers refer to this as the 72 hour bag, grab and go bag or bug out bag (BOB). These bags need to be in each vehicle and prepared for all members of the family. My main concern is nutrient dense foods. The list below will include suggestions.

There are numerous websites that will give lists of other items such as flash lights, clothing, water bottles, first aid, knives, and more that are necessary for this bag.

Imagine being on the highway and exits are at least 10 miles in both directions when a tractor trailer jack knifes and blocks all traffic in both directions. This can cause a 4-10 hour unplanned stop in the car. Alone this is tragic but with kids it can be more devastating. Everyone will get hungry and thirsty. So being prepared with these bags in each vehicle will prevent an unnecessary discomfort. Food and water plus a first aid kit are mandatory in each of our vehicles.

This is one step that needs to be completed as soon as possible.

72 Hours

First we need 72 hours of instant food. Assume there is no heat or cooking source.

Here are some options that will satisfy hunger and supply the needs of the body:

- Water bottles or a water bottle filter such as the Life Straw or the Berkie Water Bottle Filter
- Tuna and salmon in foil packages- single serve; Pack with crackers
- Granola bars
- Nut butter- single serve packets
- Protein bars; protein powders that can be mixed in water
- Dried beef jerky
- Dried trail mix
- M & M's (Yes I know these are not healthy but when dealing with trouble it may keep the family happy.)

Easy place to pick up quick food is at hotel breakfast bars. They have honey packets and peanut butter individual servings.

Have a supply of these foods in a back pack in each vehicle and in a 'quick to grab bag' at home. If the car breaks down this will keep everyone satisfied so they can think and be smart about the situation.

Practice

Practice is simple for this category; get the bags ready now and use them as needed. Remember to replace any items used so the bag is always ready. I keep a post-it note pad with a pen in each bag to write a reminder of what needs to be replaced.

Conclusion

Preparing for one week, one month or one year will be simple. Now that the inventory and list of favorites is completed, we can put together a rotating menu plan that will take the anxiety out of cooking during unusual circumstances. Keep this menu and inventory list handy near the food so that it can be referred to as needed.

Remember:

**When Momma's in control and happy
the family is in control and happy.
We can do this.**

Cooking

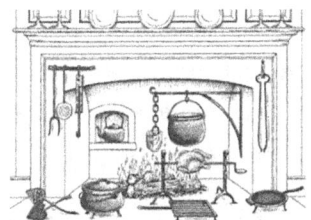

*She **rises** also while it is still night,
and **gives** food to her household,
and portions to her maidens.*

Food is not optional. If we want to be strong and healthy we must eat well. Feeding our families well means knowing how to shop, prepare and cook. There are numerous options when it comes to cooking especially when times may not be *normal*. From this list I recommend picking at least 3 ways to be prepared. Some options are for short term emergencies and others are for long term 'no power' emergencies.

Short Term Options

This means having on hand different cooking stoves or supplies for a short term need such as a power outage from a storm. Having these options on hand can also make it simpler as we perfect the other methods.

Butane Counter Top Range: These average $14 – $25 and use cans of butane as the fuel. They are simple to use and because they work with butane

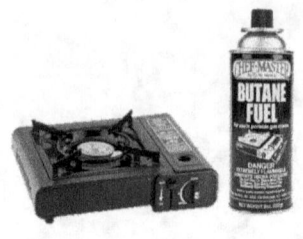

and these are safe indoors. The burner will cook like a stove. There are other options available such as two burners and more. Plus they come in pretty colors (I wish I had known before I bought mine). I use these for cooking classes at our Flavor of Grace Conferences. They are very handy and store in a nice hard case.

Most important note on this Butane Range – butane can be stored indefinitely. This means the small canisters can be stocked up for emergencies.

Gas Camping Stove: There are hundreds of options on line and in the stores. IN fact, there is probably one on your patio or in the garage. Small table top styles can easily be used indoors or out. When using these indoors good ventilation is a necessity. Many people open a window for air flow.

Kitchen Stove: The burners on a gas kitchen stove can be used without electricity by lighting with a match. The ovens generally cannot be used. Check the owner's manual.

Outdoor Gas Grill: Outdoor grills using bottled gas is an easy option. Most insurance policies will allow one extra filled gas tank in storage on the property without negating the homeowner's policy.

Convert Outdoor Gas Grills to Charcoal: Changing a gas outdoor grill to burn charcoal is a relatively easy process. (Various websites with instructions claim this to be true.)

Here are the instructions:
1. Disconnect the propane cylinder from the grill and remove all gas hoses and regulator valves from below the grill. Removal techniques will vary based on the grill type and manufacturer; having the original grill manual on hand for direction can help in this process.
2. **Leave all gas burners intact inside the grill. These will form supports for a homemade charcoal grate.**
3. Turn all gas burners to high-heat settings and open the grill lid to allow any gas remaining in the lines or burners to escape.

4. Remove the cooking grate for now and set it aside.
5. Cut chicken wire to fit the dimensions of the grill interior. This homemade charcoal grate should touch all grill walls while sitting atop the old burners inside the grill. It will provide separation between lit coals and the grill floor so oxygen can reach the heat source.
6. Drill six holes (if not already present) straight through the grill floor and between the burners to allow air from outside the grill to circulate inside. This provides an oxygen source to fan charcoal fires.
7. Place the cooking grate back into the grill.http://www.ehow.com/how_5727759_convert-gas-grill-charcoal.html

Charcoal Grills

It is recommended to have at least 120 pounds of charcoal stored per month of cooking. Watch for holiday sales such as Memorial Day, July 4th and Labor Day.

Fire

Fire and I have met under dire circumstances. In fact, I have the scars and stories as proof. Rule for fire: kerosene is safer than gasoline for starting fires. It is less explosive. Yes, that is what I learned.

For short term or evening fun around the campfire, cooking on a fire in the back yard works. A trendy fire pit with a flat grilling surface will be necessary. These trendy fire pits can be installed simply.

The pit needs to be dug at least 18 inches deep in the ground and preferably 4-5 feet in diameter. The bottom of the pit can be filled with rock or quick Crete. Then surround the dug out pit with a wall 18 inches high (above the ground level) using landscaping stones or concrete blocks as a barrier to the heat and to place the grill top on. I can see this more for roasting marshmallows and family time rather than for preparing a meal. But still, it is an option.

Long Term Options

Wood Stove - Build a more permanent wood cooking stove outdoors or buy an old fashioned one for installing indoors. Since wood is sustainable this would be both a short and long term solution.

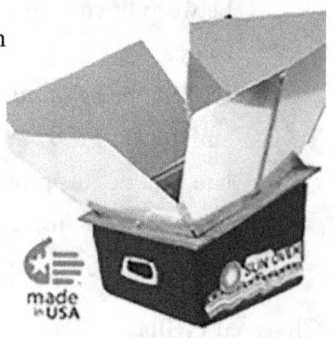

Each of these previous options so far has been common place. Let me suggest a not so common idea – Sun cooking. As I researched cooking options when there is little or no power my curiosity landed on the Sun Oven. As I studied the idea I learned an oven could be handmade with a box and foil or I could just purchase one. So I went for the simple – buy it.

When it arrived I made cookies and spaghetti, in that order. Priorities will always be important.

When the sun oven box is placed facing the sun it immediately begins heating up. Right away the temperature began climbing on the thermometer inside from 100° to 150° to 250° and up.

Imagine cooking regular favorite foods without heating up the home in the summer and not requiring any power source or charcoal. It's a sweet deal.

Even my homemade freshly milled flour bread was delicious in the Sun Oven.

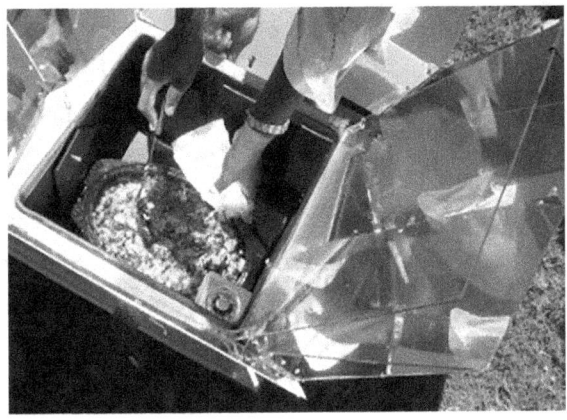

Benefits of cooking in a *SUN OVEN*®

Cook for free
Bakes, Boils or Steams Any Kind of Food with the Power of the Sun – No Fuel Needed!

No learning curve
Create your favorite recipes as you feast upon natural sun baked treats!

Just like your home oven reaches Temperatures of 360° to 400° F!

Totally Safe – No Danger of Fire – Never Burn Dinner Again!

Versatile, Easy-to-use, Portable as a Small Suitcase!

Satisfaction Guarantee: If you are not completely satisfied with your *SUN OVEN*® you may return it within 30 days of the date you receive it and you will receive a refund. What are you waiting for?

Cooking in a *SUN OVEN* is easy, fun, natural, and nutritious. *SUN OVENS* are ideal for everyday use in your back yard, at picnics, while camping, or in the event of a power failure. They can help keep your house cool in the summer by keeping the heat from cooking outside.

Even though it is called an oven, food can be baked, boiled and steamed at cooking temperatures of 360° F to 400° F. There is no movement of air in a *SUN OVEN*®, allowing food to stay moist and tender and flavorful. Sun-baked roasts are tastier and more succulent, and sunbaked bread has unparalleled taste and texture. The aroma of food sunning itself in a *SUN OVEN*® is sure to please your senses.

There are two ways to cook in a *SUN OVEN*®. If you refocus the oven to follow the sun every 25 to 30 minutes, cooking times and methods will be very similar to cooking with a conventional stove or oven. Or a *SUN OVEN*® can be used for slow cooking, much like a crock-pot. You can prepare your dinner, put it in the *SUN OVEN*®, point the oven where the sun will be approximately halfway through the time you will be gone. Leave, and come home to a tasty, slow-cooked dinner. If you run late, there is no need to worry; the *SUN OVEN*® will keep your food warm, moist, and fresh for hours.

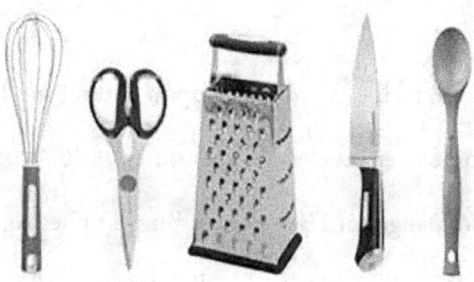

Kitchen Supplies

It is never fun to cook without the necessary utensils. When I was a young bride over 33 years ago I loved using all the new gadgets and gifts from the bridal showers and wedding gifts. But as the years go by so does the newness of the gifts. Utensils get lost, broken or worn out. If times may get more difficult then I want to have the necessities.

Here is a list of my "Must-Have's" in the kitchen:
- Liquid and dry measuring cups
- Measuring spoons – I love the stainless steel

- Thermometer – both oven and cooking for meats and breads
- Canning set – this is a 6 piece canning set of utensils that will be talked about in the canning section. I cooked without them for years to avoid spending the $12. They are worth every penny.
- Wooden spoons – these spoons continue to be essential because of their usefulness for mixing and stirring either in a bowl or in a pot on the stove. They are also ideal for use in nonstick cookware.
- Ladle
- Spatula
- Tongs
- Slotted spoons
- Whisk
- Knives: chef's, serrated bread knife, paring knife and knife sharpener
- Garlic press
- Grater
- Potato masher
- Hand operated can opener
- Timer
- Vegetable Peeler
- Colanders – preferably with footed bottom
- Kitchen shears
- Cutting boards
- Vegetable scrubbing brush
- Rolling pin
- Dough scraper
- Pastry blender
- Cutting Boards

Appliances

Having the right appliances will make cooking fun. The first list is my powered appliances and the second is for when there is no power.

Electric Appliances
- *Mock Mill - for milling grains, beans, non-oi
- Mini Nutrimill – for milling spices, flax seed
- *Bosch Mixer with meat grinder, cookie paddl
- Immersion Blender – not necessary until yo won't want to be without!
- Food Processor
- *Blender – high powered like the Bosch Blender, Vita Mix or other similar
- *Dehydrator

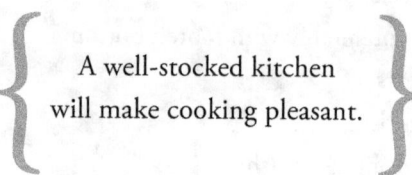

Non-Power Appliances
- *Hand mill – for milling grains, beans, seeds, etc.
- Slice & Grate – hand powered quick slicer and grater
- Sauce master – perfect for making sauces and purees
- Mini battery powered blender
- Can opener
- Apple peeler, corer and slicer
- Hand crank for Bosch Mixer

{ A well-stocked kitchen will make cooking pleasant. }

Cookware
- *Good quality pots and pans: Stainless steel, cast iron, crockery
- *Bakeware
- *Bread pans
- Canner – water bath canner
- *Pressure Canner (can also be the water bath canner)
- *Must have.

Conclusion

Pray about this cooking material.

Plan - What are three types of cooking methods that seem doable for your situation?

Put Into Action – What cooking appliances and utensils are needed in the kitchen for these cooking options to be implemented?

Practice – Practice these cooking methods at least weekly to stay comfortable with the tools and situations.

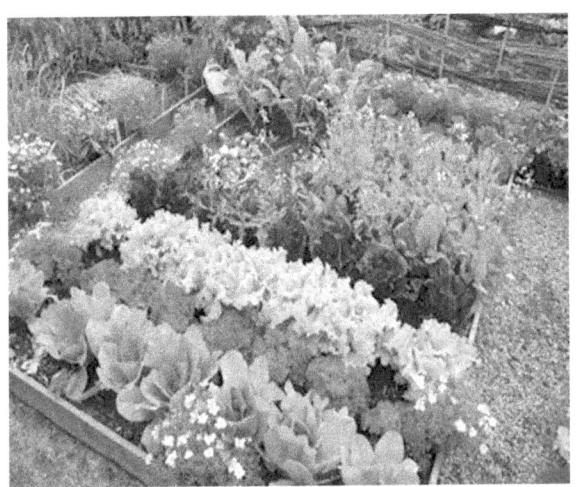

Gardening

Stocking shelves with food will carry us through difficult storms and yes, many people are stocking up a year's worth of food. But if I can garden I stretch my budget and save on storage needs. And who doesn't want fresh food versus canned? So learning how to garden will enrich your meals and delight your palates.

As a child, my dad, who grew up on the farm, would plant this humongous garden in our yard. Rows and rows of vegetables all summer long we had to weed, pick, chop, weed, pick, chop, and weed. You get the picture. Even though I loved to eat, I detested working so hard to put it on the table. I admit, I wasn't the most pleasant child when it came to forced labor.

Now today, I start my mornings walking through the garden. I can't wait to see the action happening. When will the berries be ready to eat? What's happening under the soil? When will my harvest come in? I love getting my hands dirty. In fact in the summer my nail color is brown. I am almost in style!

Gardening today is more than just tilling up a plot of ground. There are several options; consider which one is best for you.

In my yard the jury is still out on that answer and I have tried all types. My visitors will find raised beds, wood chip gardening, container gardening and sometimes indoor gardening.

> She considers a field and buys it, from her earnings she plants a vineyard.

Let's review each one.

Raised Bed Gardening – aka Square Foot Gardening

Mel Bartholomew has popularized this type of gardening with his book *The Square Foot Garden*. The idea is to raise the beds, fill them with the perfect mix of nutrients, feed with compost and plant to your heart's and stomach's desire. Need more food – add more beds. They are ideal for rotating crops, planting three times a year in the same location and best of all for me – it is impossible to overwater.

In one of my first beds I decided to plant a couple white sweet potato slips. I had never planted sweet potatoes before, so how hard can they be? But my curiosity was getting the best of me. I prefer planting food I can see growing such as tomatoes or blueberries. But with sweet potatoes – flowers like morning glories are visible but food is not. Many days I would try to push the dirt away and see if there was anything underneath. Then finally, in October I started reaching into the dirt. I pulled out a small potato. Well, that was good. Then I reached in again and this time the potato was as long as my forearm. Now that was really good. I kept this up, digging with my hands and arms till I was deep into the soil and pulling up potato after potato. When I finished I had two bushels of organic white sweet potatoes from just 2 potato slips. My square foot garden had delivered on its promises.

No shovel? Yes, the square foot garden does not get packed down; it is still light and airy. So I was able to harvest my potatoes with just my hands.

Benefits:
- More food in less space
- Plant three seasons
- Anyone can do it in any space

Wood Chip Gardening

Our back yard used to be small and surrounded by woods. Then I learned about wood chip gardening. We hired a tree expert and he cleared our trees back 30 feet. Next we had fresh cut wood chips hauled in for us to cover the newly exposed land with 5-6 inches of these chips. Voila! – a new garden space rich with decomposed trees, humus and topped with fresh wood chips.

In the woods the trees that have fallen decay. These decaying trees and plants create a rich humus soil. This is perfectly rich soil for growing a garden.

This environment can be created simply. First remove the grass as much as possible. Then add a layer of cardboard so that the grass or weeds don't grow up. On top of that add 5-6 inches of good dirt mixed with compost. Then add the 'icing' for the garden which is the layer of wood chips. Make the wood chips layer at least 4 inches deep. As these chips break down over the year they will add humus to the soil and become a fertilizer for the garden.

Container Gardening

Almost anything can be grown in a container. Add them to your patios, balconies, driveways and more. Any sized container that fits the space can be used to grow food. Keep In mind a few things:

- Many things can be used as a container, just make sure it is big enough for a full grown plant and that it didn't contain any chemicals that are harmful. Wash, recycle and reuse.
- Containers dry out more quickly than in ground plantings; the heat of summer may require watering twice a day.
- If the containers are on concrete, the reflective heat will make the surrounding environment much hotter than if planted in the ground.
- They need to be fertilized and amended each planting cycle.
- Hanging baskets are a great way to increase space. Some vegetable varieties thrive when grown this way.

Here is a quick list of growing in containers.

Name	Size of container	Inches between seeds	Notes
Beans	2 gal.	2-3	45-60 days to harvest
Beets	½ gal	6-8 inches	50-60 days to harvest
Carrots	1 quart	2-3 inches	50 days to harvest
Cabbage	5 gal.	12-18 inches	65-120 days, needs fertile soil
Chard, Swiss	½ gal.	4-6 inches	30-40 days to harvest
Cucumbers	5 gal.	14-18 inches	70-80 days require hot weather
Eggplant	5 gal.	1 plant per bucket	75-100 days to harvest, fertile soil
Kale	5 gal.	1 plant	Harvest leaves
Lettuce	½ gal.	4-6 inches	Harvest leaves
Mustard greens	½ gal.	4-5 inches	35-40 days to harvest

Name	Size of container	Inches between seeds	Notes
Onions	½ gal.	2-3 inches	Require lots of moisture
Peppers	2 gal.	1 plant	110-120 days to harvest, requires hot weather
Radishes	1 pint	1 plant	25-35 days to harvest
Squash, summer	5 gal.	1 plant	50-60 days
Tomatoes	5 gal.	1 plant	55-110 days to harvest
Turnips	3 gal.	2-3 inches	30-60 days to harvest leaves and roots

Indoor Gardening

With a sunny window and/or grow lights a harvest of lettuce, herbs, sprouts, some vegetables and potatoes can be enjoyed all year long.

My experience with potatoes outside in my raised bed made me very curious if I could grow these indoors as well. This past year I took my potatoes purchased from the store and rooted them in a jar in the window. It worked beautifully. Then to grow them indoors, all I needed was a large 5 gallon bucket or similar depth container and grow lights.

Potatoes are filling and satisfying. So learning to grow them in our homes can save a lot of money.

Seed storing

Having our own seeds is important when preparing to feed our families. Most recommended is the heirloom or open pollinated so another crop can be produced resulting seeds. Hybrid seeds do not repopulate. So a sustainable, long-term solution should include heirloom seeds from which seeds can be saved for the following season.

Following are some simple directions on how to save seed from some of the most commonly grown garden vegetables:
(http://aggie-horticulture.tamu.edu/archives/parsons/vegetables/SEED.html)

BEANS (all kinds)- Allow the seed to thoroughly mature on the plant, usually indicated by size of the seed in the pod or by the color of the pod. Pull the entire plant early in the morning and place it in the shade to dry out. This will prevent the pods from splitting open and the beans from shattering.

CUCUMBERS - Cross pollination occurs in cucumbers. This means pollen is transferred from a plant of one variety to a plant of another variety. This is done by insects. Although it does not affect the fruit borne this season, the seed saved and planted next year will produce different plants and fruit. So, when saving cucumber seed, plant only one variety. Select strong, healthy cucumber plants and well-formed fruits. Let the fruits hang on the vine until ripe (skin becomes yellowish and hard). Then handle like the process for tomatoes given below.

EGGPLANT - When the eggplant fruit has obtained maximum size and shows some evidence of browning and shriveling, it is ready to be harvested for seed. Split open, remove the seed and wash thoroughly to remove all pulp. Spread out in the sun to dry quickly as moist seed will begin to germinate overnight if left in a damp condition. Store in a cool, dry place.

OKRA - Okra pods should be left on the stalk until brown and well matured. Remove the pods and place them in the shade until thoroughly dried. Although the seed may be removed from the pod, it is generally best to store them in the pod until ready for planting at which time the pods may be split open and the seed removed. Pods harvested too green will not store well and are likely to split, shattering the seed.

PEPPERS - Pepper should be allowed to ripen until they become red. Cut the pepper pod in half and scrape the seed from a cavity onto a piece of paper. Spread out the seed and dry thoroughly before placing in a storage container.

SOUTHERN PEAS - Southern peas should be left on the plant until thoroughly matured, usually indicated by a browning of the pods. The pods should be picked, spread out in a dry area and cured for a week or two, then shelled.

SQUASH - If seed are to be saved from squash, grow only one variety in the garden. When the outer covering of the squash has become hardened, the seed are generally mature. Split the squash fruit open, scoop out the seed and wash until all pulp is removed. Spread out on newspaper to dry.

TOMATOES - Allow the tomato fruit to thoroughly ripen on the vine. Cut the tomatoes open and remove the seed by squeezing or spooning out the pulp with seeds into a non-metal container such as a drinking glass or jar. Set the container aside for one or two days. The pulp and seed covering will ferment so that the seeds can be washed clean with a directed spray of water into the fermented solution. The clean, viable seeds will drop to the bottom of the solution, allowing the sediment to pour off. Several rinses may be necessary. Then spread the tomato seed out on a cloth or paper towel to dry. After seeds are dry; package, label and date for storage in a cool (refrigerator), dry location.

Herb Seeds

Keep herbs in mind when planning a garden. Many herbs are perennials and will come back the next year without replanting, depending on your climate. In my garden are oregano, sage and spearmint. They continue to spread and add to the beauty of my gardenHerbs are typically easy to grow, add nutrition and flavor to your meals, and they dehydrate and store readily.

Sprouting Seeds

And don't forget sprouting seeds! Sprouts are extremely nutritious and versatile and very easy to grow indoors in just a few days. During an emergency time, sprouts offer a lot of nutrition in a small amount of food. Sprouts have higher protein, fiber and enzymes than the original seed. This benefits the body with the microbiome being more protective against parasites and also boost the immune system.

There are many different sprouts to choose from as well. The most common sprout that you'll likely see in the grocery store is alfalfa. But there is also red clover, broccoli, and others. Wheat grains and dried beans like lentils make tasty sprouts as well.

Sprouting the Jar-Lid Method
This is the simplest and cheapest method for sprouting. Any standard wide-mouth jar can be used together with a sprouting screen, sprouting jar lid or a small piece of tulle and a rubber band.

- **Directions:**
- Place 1-2 Tablespoons sprouting seeds in a clean wide-mouth jar.
- Place the sprouting screen and ring, sprout lid or tulle and rubber band over the top of the jar. The green leaves is a sign the sprouts are ready to eat.
- Fill the jar with water and then pour off to rinse seed.
- Fill jar with water and let soak for 4-12 hours, depending on the type of sprouts.
- Drain water, then rinse with water twice each day for 5 days until sprouts are finished.
- Store sprout jar in a bowl, tilted at an angle so any excess water drains out through the screen. Sprouts should be moist, not sitting in water.
- Once sprouts have grown to be an inch or so long and have formed very small leaves called cotyledons, the sprouts are ready for greening. Just place the jar in bright indirect light and they will turn green over the course of a day.

Enjoy fresh sprouts on sandwiches, salads and more!

Store sprouts in the refrigerator for up to a week. If not stored in an airtight container, rinse sprouts with water each day to keep them moist.

Conclusion

Pray about how to add fresh garden foods to your menu.

Plan - What are two types of gardening methods that seem doable for your situation? Is there someone you know who will allow others to garden on their property?

Put Into Action – What gardening implements are needed for gardening?

Practice – Practice gardening, working with tools, and digging in the dirt. All homes or apartments can at least grow herbs on the window sill.

Bottom line for gardening…..
Grow what you love, love what you grow!

Preserving Food

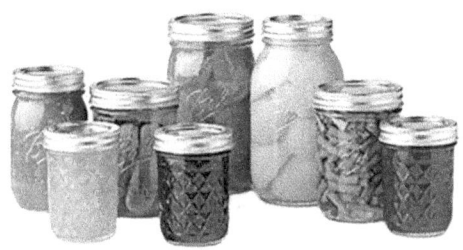

Nutritious and tasty are the exact words to describe foods that will come from the kitchen as these preserving skills are perfected.

When I was shown a jar of canned deer meat several years ago I thought I was back in lab class looking at a jar of organs in formaldehyde. No, I was not going to eat that. But the quickest way for me to change my opinion was by actually tasting it. So, hesitantly, I tried my first bite. Let me say it was "melt-in-your-mouth" good. This meant I must learn how to do it.

{ She looks well to the ways of her household and does not eat the bread of idleness. }

Let me first share a really good website for most questions and answers: www.pickyourown.org. There is no need to buy books when this website will teach everything necessary to try this process. Plus this link on their site will give the crop harvest calendar for each state: http://pickyourown.org/US_crop_harvest_calendars.php

Here are some quick charts of the basics of each process.

Knowing how to do each one will be helpful since different foods require different processes.

Water-Bath Canning
Storage time: Suggested 2-5 years

Supplies Needed
- Big canning pot (can be a pressure canner)
- Rack – or towel if rack is not available
- Jar lifter
- Jar funnel
- Jars, lids, and rings to hold lids on

Perfect For:
- Jams, jellies, and preserves
- Fruit
- Applesauce
- Pickles
- Tomato products

Steps
1. Gather supplies and equipment.
2. Keep jars hot (I do this in the canner water).
3. Prepare food.
4. Fill jars, leaving proper headspace and releasing air bubbles. Put on lids and hand-tighten screw bands.
5. Place jars in water-bath canner.
6. Cover jars with 1-2 inches of water.
7. Bring water to boil and allow boiling for amount of time specified in recipe.
8. At end of processing time, remove jars and allow to cool completely.
9. Test seals.

10. Store!
11. Enjoy – yes, it is art and looks beautiful on the shelf, but eating is what it was meant for.

Steam Pressure Canning
Storage time: Suggested 2-5 years

Supplies Needed
- Pressure Canner with valves, seals, and gauges
- Rack
- Jar lifter
- Jar funnel
- Jars, lids, and rings to hold lids on

Perfect For:
- Vegetables
- Meat
- Butter – made into ghee
- Soups
- Plus almost everything that can be done as water bath canning can be pressure canned.

Steps
1. Gather supplies and equipment; keep jars hot.
2. Prepare food.
3. Fill jars, leaving proper headspace and releasing air bubbles. Put on lids and hand-tighten screw bands.
4. Place jars in pressure canner.
5. Close and lock the canner.
6. Process jars as outlined in the recipe.
7. At end of processing time, allow pressure to return to 0.
8. Remove jars from canner and allow to cool completely.
9. Test seals.
10. Store!

Freezing
Storage time: 2 months – 1 year

Supplies Needed
- Food to store
- Freezer bags
- Vacuum Sealer - optional

Perfect For:
Almost anything

Not – Perfect For:
- Canned food
- Eggs in shells
- Lettuce greens
- Summer squash - raw

Steps:
1. Gather supplies.
2. Prepare food.
3. Place food in freezer containers, leaving specified headspace (if using rigid containers) or pressing out all excess air (if using freezer storage bags).
4. Slightly chill food or, if it was blanched, allow to come to room temperature.
5. Loosely pack food in freezer.
6. When completely frozen, repack more tightly in freezer.

For fruits, I like to do a quick freeze on a cookie sheet in the freezer before placing them in freezer bags. This allows me to remove them individually when they are totally frozen.

Hints: Freezer burn does not make food unsafe, merely dry in spots. It appears as grayish-brown leathery spots and is caused by air reaching the surface of the food. Cut freezer-burned portions away either before or after cooking the food. Heavily freezer-burned foods may have to be discarded for quality reasons.

Blanching slows or stops the action of enzymes which cause loss of flavor, color and texture. Blanching cleanses the surface of dirt and organisms, brightens the color and helps retard loss of vitamins. Blanching also wilts or softens vegetable and makes them easier to pack.

Vegetables should be cooled quickly and thoroughly after blanching to stop the cooking process. Otherwise, vegetables will be overcooked with loss of flavor, color, vitamins and minerals.

Adjustments for High-Altitude Canning

Home cooks who live at high altitudes may be used to adjusting recipes; high-altitude adjustments apply to home canning, as well. Canning food safely requires filled jars to be processed at a specified temperature or pressure level for a specified amount of time. At altitudes higher than 1,000 or 2,000 feet above sea level, adjust the canning recipes for food safety.

- **Water-bath canning:** Generally, recipes are written for water bath canning at altitudes less than 1000 feet. If you live higher than 1,000 feet above sea level, follow these guidelines:

  For processing times of less than 20 minutes: Add 1 additional minute for each additional 1000 feet of altitude.

  For processing times of more than 20 minutes: Add 2 additional minutes for each 1000 feet of altitude.

- **Pressure Canning:** Pressure canning recipes are generally written for altitudes of less than 2000 feet. For those living higher than 2000 feet above sea level, make this adjustment: Increase pounds of pressure by ½ pound for each additional 1,000 feet.

Tips for Successful and Safe Canning

Keep safety in mind whether water-bath canning or steam pressure canning. By canning foods safely, kitchen accidents and food spoilage can be prevented. Increase your chances for successful canning and maximum safety by following these guidelines:

- Use recipes made for modern-day canning (about year 2000 or newer) and follow them exactly. Don't increase or decrease ingredients, processing time, or pressure level (for pressure canning).

- Don't double recipes. Prepare the recipes more than once; do not double the ingredients.

- Use the proper ingredients: only unblemished and not overly ripe fruit or vegetables, and when a recipe calls for salt, use only canning or pickling salt.

- Use jars and two-piece lids approved for canning, and never reuse lids.

- Always label and date the finished product.

- Periodically check jars for any signs of spoilage and, if in doubt about the quality or safety of a preserved product, dispose of it without tasting.

Dehydrating
Storage time: Suggested up to 1 year

Supplies Needed
- Good sharp knife
- A spatula or two
- Dehydrator
- And these items are helpful:
- Food processor
- Apple peeler-slicer-corer
- Blender for pureeing
- Strainer

Perfect for:
Almost everything including vegetables, fruit, breads, cooked ground meat, granola, brownies, and the list continues.

Easy way to not let food go bad. If you have small bits of extra vegetables or fruits – dehydrate them for a soup or dessert later.

Steps:
1. Gather supplies.
2. Prepare food.
3. Arrange food on dehydrator trays.
4. Dry at specified temperature, occasionally turning food and rotating trays.
5. Check for doneness, using guidelines in recipe for what properly dried food looks and feels like.
6. Place in airtight storage container and store in cool, dry place out of direct sunlight.

Top 2 Dehydrators

LeQuip Filter Pro Dehydrator – this machine I love because it has an air filter to make sure the air going across the food is clean and filtered. It also has stacking trays that can go up to 20 high. I only use the main 6. They come in two depths for different size cuts of food. It also has a timer and LED temperature. The timer allows me to leave the process. I love this option since I can be gone over 10 hours or want it to finish during the night.

Excalibur - this is the second most popular. I used this in our video series. It is highly praised but since I have experienced both I love the Filter Pro much better. The new Excalibur's are drying with the same mechanics as the Lequip

Both are very good options. There are cheaper options in the store and of course dehydrating can be done in the oven or sun on a hot day.

Freeze Dried
Storage Time: 25 years

Freeze Dried foods can be done in the home but only with the freeze drying oven. When I priced them they were $3,000. No, that is not in my budget. So where to turn?

Freeze dried foods are found in several different web stores. The food will keep up to 25 years and is incredibly tastier than dehydrated or canned.

Typically freeze dried or vacuum packed is sold in 10# cans and the cost will vary from $10 up to $40 depending on the food included. My concerns with this type of food are the quality. Most of it is shipping in from China and the inspection of these foods is nominal if at all.

When buying this food look for these important tips:

> Buy American
> Buy only non-GMO foods
> Buy only the foods you know you love
> Never buy TVP – it is always GMO soy beans

Tools and Equipment for Canning and Preserving
If you plan to can, freeze, or dry your food, you'll need some special tools. The equipment involved with canning or preserving food is designed for efficiency and safety. If you have these pieces already, great! If not, add them to your shopping list:

- **Tongs:** Have tongs ready for lifting hot foods out of boiling or simmering water. Any variety will work, but a locking mechanism keeps them out of the way when not in use.
- **Candy thermometer:** Find a good quality thermometer, with a clip for attaching it to the side of a pot. This item is so useful; it is a good idea to have a backup in case one breaks during use.
- **Jar lifter:** This tool is a specialized set of tongs. Its rubberized ends fit securely around any size canning jar, to lift them in and out of the canner.

- **Canning funnel:** Used for canning foods, this wide mouth tool keeps the rims of jars clean. It can also be used to fill Ziploc bags neatly.
- **Canning jars:** Canning jars are made from tempered glass to withstand the high heat and pressure of a canner. Both narrow- and wide-mouth jars are available, with wide-mouth being easiest to remove the food from once it is canned.
- **Water-bath and/or pressure canner.** If canning, use the appropriate canner. For canning high-acid foods (fruits, jellies, relishes, and pickles), get a water-bath canner. For low-acid foods (vegetables and meats), get a pressure canner.

Root Cellars

Root cellars are more than a location; they are a storage method. To keep this book from being an encyclopedia I suggest further research of this topic.

Food can easily be stored in the most unlikely places if prepared correctly. Imagine a trash can buried in the yard or storing food in the crawl space. Yes – sounds weird, but when it comes to maintaining a healthy abundance of highly nutritious foods this is an option not to overlook.

Loss of Power

Does the word *Isabel* bring memories back? When we first moved into our home in Richmond the next weekend our first hurricane experience happened. *Isabel.* Moving here from the mid-west a hurricane was a new experience. After the storm passed our neighborhood came alive. Everyone brought out the grills and started having a huge barbeque since the freezers were now without power. There were many people in Richmond without power for over 6-10 weeks.

Since a power loss affects the frozen and refrigerated foods there are ways to better prepare for this situation.

First – pack the freezer full. When my freezer is not full of food then I fill it with water bottles or frozen milk cartons filled with water. Let there be no space not filled. A full freezer will remain frozen 24 hours longer than a half empty freezer.

Second – when there is an expectation that the power will be out in the home, immediately set the temperature at a lower (colder) level. This will delay thawing. Preferably this is done at least 24 hours in advance for the refrigerator/freezer to compensate.

Dry ice can also be used.

A fully- loaded freezer at 0° will stay cold enough to keep frozen foods frozen for 2-3 days. A freezer half-filled may not keep frozen food frozen for more than one day.

Do not open the freezer or refrigerator door while the power is off.

If power is going to be off for longer than 2-3 days then this food is the first choice for eating. If there is enough power or gas, the food can be canned in the pressure canner on a gas grill.

Using a generator for the freezer and refrigerator is also a good option. Solar generators can provide power without the need for gas.

Conclusion

Pray about these preserving methods.

Plan - What are at least two types of preserving methods that seem doable?

Put Into Action – What appliances and utensils are needed in the kitchen for these preserving options to be implemented?

Practice – Practice these preserving methods. I suggest learning each one and then start using what seems comfortable. Trade or barter with others who use other methods.

Recipes

Ready for Fun with Dehydrating?
This is taking dehydrating to a new fun level; plus… think of the Christmas and Bridal Shower gifts which can be prepared.

These recipes are from *The Complete Dehydrator Coobook*

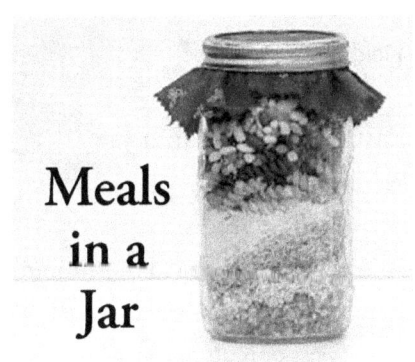

Meals in a Jar

Beef Barley Soup Mix in a Jar
- 1 (1 pint) jar
- ¾ cup medium pearl barley, separated
- ½ cup dried lentils
- 2 tablespoons dried parsley flakes
- ¼ cup dried minced onions
- ¼ cup instant beef bouillon
- 2 tablespoons dried celery flakes
- ½ teaspoon dried thyme leaves
- 2 bay leaves
- ¼ teaspoon black pepper
- ¼ teaspoon dried minced garlic

Layer soup kit ingredients in jar in order listed, using half of barley first and then remaining barley at the top. Close jar securely with lid. Attach cooking instructions (below).

Beef Barley Soup

1   (2 pound) boneless beef chuck, cut in ½- to ¾-inch pieces or 2 pound lean hamburger (options: canned meat or dehydrated meat)
1   tablespoon oil
    Contents of gift jar
10 cups water

Heat oil in Dutch oven over medium heat and brown the meat. Pour off drippings. Add the contents of soup kit jar and water to Dutch oven; bring to a boil. Reduce heat; cover tightly and simmer 1½ to 1¾ hours or until beef is fork tender.

Discard bay leaves.

Yields 8 servings.

Pasta Soup Mix in a Jar

½   cup macaroni
¼   cup dried lentils
¼   cup dried, chopped mushrooms
2   tablespoons Parmesan cheese, grated
1   tablespoon onion flakes
1   tablespoon chicken soup base
1   teaspoon dried parsley
½   teaspoon oregano
1   dash garlic powder

Mix Parmesan cheese, onion flakes, soup base, parsley, oregano and garlic powder together in a small bowl.

In a one pint jar, layer ingredients in this order:

Spice mixture
Macaroni
Lentils
Mushrooms

Store with tightly sealed lid, until needed.

Attach the following recipe with a hang tag to give as a gift:

Basic Pasta Soup

Combine contents of jar with 3 cups water in a 2 quart saucepan. Bring to a boil, then reduce heat. Cover and simmer for 40 minutes or until lentils are tender, stirring occasionally.

Makes 4 servings.

Country Soup Mix in a Jar

Fills one 1-quart jar

- ½ cup barley
- ½ cup dried split peas
- ½ cup uncooked rice
- ½ cup dry lentils
- 2 tablespoons dried minced onion
- 2 tablespoons dried parsley
- 2 teaspoons salt
- ½ teaspoon lemon pepper
- 2 tablespoons beef bouillon granules
- ½ cup uncooked alphabet pasta
- 1 cup uncooked twist macaroni

In a wide mouth 1-quart jar, layer the barley, peas, rice and lentils. Then layer around the edges the onion, parsley, salt, lemon pepper, bouillon and the alphabet pasta. Fill the rest of the jar with the twist macaroni. Seal.

Attach a gift card with the following instructions:

Country Soup

Add contents of jar to 3 quarts of water, 2 stalks chopped celery, 2 sliced carrots, 1 cup shredded cabbage (optional) and 2 cups diced tomatoes. Over medium low heat, cover and simmer about 1 hour, or until vegetables are tender.

The celery, carrots, cabbage and tomatoes can be dehydrated and saved in a sealed package to accompany this recipe.

Potato Soup Mix in a Jar

- 1¾ cups dehydrated hash potatoes
- 1½ cups dried milk
- 2 tablespoons instant chicken bouillon
- 2 teaspoons dried minced onion
- 1 teaspoon dried parsley
- ¼ teaspoon ground white pepper
- ¼ teaspoon dried thyme
- ⅛ teaspoon turmeric
- 1½ teaspoons seasoning salt

Combine all ingredients in a bowl; mix well. Put ingredients in a 1-quart jar.

On gift tag write: Place ½ cup mix in soup bowl; add 1 cup of boiling water; stir until smooth.

Taco Bean Chili Mix in a Jar

- ½ cup dried kidney beans
- ½ cup dried pinto beans
- ½ cup dried red beans
- 1 (1¼ ounce) package taco seasoning mix (or your own mixture of spices)
- 1 tablespoon dried minced onion
- ½ teaspoon chili powder or chipotle chili pepper seasoning
- ¼ teaspoon ground cumin
- 1½ cups tortilla chips, slightly crushed

Layer ingredients in 1-quart wide-mouth jar in following order: kidney beans, pinto beans and red beans. Place taco seasoning mix, onion, chili powder and cumin in small plastic zip-type bag. Seal bag and place bag in jar. Add tortilla chips. Seal jar.

Decorate jar and attach the following instructions on a gift tag:

Taco Bean Chili
Makes 6 to 8 servings.

1	jar Taco Bean Chili Mix
4	cups water
1	(14½ ounce) can diced tomatoes with green Chile's (Ro*Tel), undrained
1	(8 ounce) can tomato sauce
1	pound ground beef or ground turkey, browned and drained
	Shredded cheese, chopped lettuce, sliced black olives (optional)

Remove tortilla chips and seasoning packet from jar mix. Set aside.

Place beans in large bowl. Cover with water. Soak 6 to 8 hours or overnight. To quick-soak beans, place beans in large saucepan; cover with water. Bring to a boil over high heat. Boil 2 minutes. Remove from heat; let soak, covered, 1 hour. Drain beans; discard water.

Place soaked beans, water, tomatoes, tomato sauce, ground beef and contents of seasoning packet in Dutch oven. Bring to a boil over high heat. Cover. Reduce heat and simmer 1½ to 2 hours or until beans are tender.

Crush tortilla chips. Stir into chili and cook 5 to 10 minutes to thicken. Serve with cheese, lettuce and olives, if desired.

Use leftover chili to make a taco salad.

Read more at http://www.recipegoldmine.com/foodgiftsoup/taco-bean-chili.html#oXOg8OmwBFvV370w.99

Cleaning

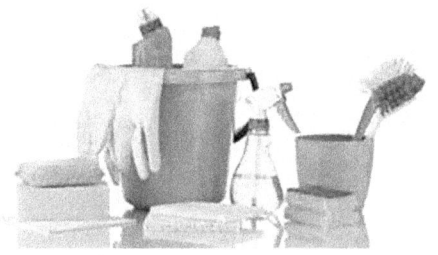

In my dreams my house never needs cleaning, but then I wake up. A clean home is a healthy home. It is ok for dirt to come in but not to stay. It is never ok for chemicals to come in.

Clean is important but not at the sacrifice of our health. Products such as 409, Tide, Lysol, etc. are toxic and cause difficulty breathing. When I work with clients with allergies and mental issues the first step taken is eliminate and replace their cleaning products. These highly toxic chemicals cause respiratory issues and a host of other seemingly non related concerns including hormonal problems. Removing these toxins will assist the body to rid itself of the toxins. That is a tough job and very rewarding.

So let's start with your home. What are you using that may be causing harm? In the *Treasures of Healthy Living Bible Study* I cover this in more detail in Week 9: Environment and Toxins.

Remember we are trying to be prepared, but if our families are sick and toxic then it will be harder to thrive under stressful situations. So while preparing let's also start repairing the immune system.

The cleaners I am going to recommend will help everyone in the family breathe better and increase their immune health.

There are hundreds of websites listing cleaning suggestions using lemons, oil, vinegar and many other ideas. They all work to a degree but for me the smell of vinegar plus the cost is a deterring factor. Yes, the recipes I list first are cheaper options than store bought cleaners but still more expensive than what I use.

To start here are some DIY cleaner recipes. These are not my favorite but I know some DIYers will like this option. Then I will follow with my favorite – simple, easy, and organic cleaners.

DIY Homemade Cleaners

Being prepared means you will already have these ingredients on hand. The mixes don't need to be premade but the ingredients on the shelf will give you peace of mind that you can do this.

Window, Floor, General Surface Cleaner

- ½ cup white vinegar – not Apple cider vinegar
- 32 oz. (1 quart) cups water
- ¼ tsp. to ½ tsp. peppermint essential oil (Mountain Rose Herbs website is a good source)

Make up a batch in a repurposed juice jug. Fill spray bottles from this master supply. Tea Tree Juice, Lemon Juice or some other scent can be added by using essential oils. Peppermint oil or tea tree oil are good for their antibacterial and antiseptic qualities.

All Purpose Cleaner

- 1 Tbsp. Dr. Bronner's Sal Suds
- 32 oz. (1 quart) cups water

Good for prewashing dishes, granite counters, removing grease off sinks, and removing spots from clothing.

Disinfecting Spray Cleaner
¼ – ½ cup Rubbing Alcohol
32 oz. (1 quart) cups water

Mix and put in sprayer. It even brightens things such as granite countertops and stainless steel.

Dirt Cheap Soft Soap or Body Wash
1   cup grated bar soap
10 cups water, preferably filtered
1   tbsp. glycerin (can be purchased from Amazon)
1 – 2 tsp essential oils, optional (Mountain Rose Herbs)

Directions:
1. Grate the soap.
2. Place the grated soap flakes into a large pot and add the water and glycerin.
3. Put the pot on the stove and turn the burner up to a medium heat. After about a minute, the flakes will dissolve. At this point whip into a heavenly, bubbly froth.
4. Set homemade soap aside to cool. Let it sit overnight or for a few hours at a minimum.
Dirt Cheap Soft Soap will get thicker as it cools. I have found that different soaps thicken differently. Some got too thick so I simply added more water the next day and whisked it up some more to blend it all together.
5. Pour this Dirt Cheap Soft Soap into containers. For each batch I used 2 re-purposed 1/2 gallon apple juice jugs as storage containers. I used a funnel which helps a lot. I then used the juice jugs to fill my counter top soap dispensers.

Better Than Good Laundry Soap

- 3 tablespoons Borax (such as Twenty Mule Team)
- 3 tablespoons Washing Soda (such as Arm & Hammer)
- 2 tablespoons Liquid Dish Soap
- 8 cups water

Directions:

Find a ½ gallon container such as a clean juice bottle that has been repurposed. Get out a funnel and add the borax and washing soda followed by 2 cups of boiling water. Give it all a good shake until the powdered ingredients are dissolved.

Add the liquid dish soap and swish it around until the brew is well mixed.

Once that is done, add the remaining water which will pretty much fill the jug. Do not be surprised if there are bubbles coming out of the top – that is the dish soap doing its thing.

When it is time to do laundry, measure out ¼ cup to ½ cup of this DIY laundry detergent and wash normally. This detergent will be thin and watery but don't worry, it will work just fine.

Drain Cleaner

- 1 cup baking soda
- 1 cup white vinegar

Hot or boiling water

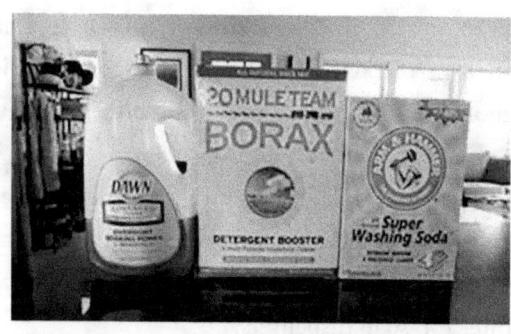

Pour the baking soda and vinegar into the drain and let it sit for an hour with the stopper down. Remove the stopper and add a kettle of really hot water (or boiling water if careful) down the drain. If used every month or so, the drain will stay nice and clear.

This works great in bathroom sinks where hair, makeup and other particles can quickly create pesky clogs.

Toilet Bowl Cleaner
Inspired by livesimply.me

- 1 cup boiled water, cooled
- ½ cup Baking Soda
- ½ cup Castile Soap
    - Favorite essential oil drops for aroma
    - Vinegar with spray top

Add the water, baking soda, castile soap and essential oil drops to a squirt bottle and shake. Save vinegar till ready to clean.

To clean: Squirt the mixed toilet bowl cleaner in the toilet bowl, scrub the toilet and then spray straight with the vinegar. Allow the vinegar to sit for 5 minutes for a thorough disinfectant.

These recipes are from:
Livesimply.me
Backdoorsurvival.com

Now for the Easy - Organic – Simple Solution
Home should be the safest place on earth. Clean with products that are safe, powerful and green.

Here are two companies that offer this solution.

Branch Basics is my new favorite company. I have been using their products for a year and they far outshine all competitors. A basic product that can be used multiple ways.

Replace dozens of toxic cleaners with one Concentrate that can do it all. The bottles are refillable so they're better for the environment and your wallet! The ingredients in Branch Basics (which is very transparent) includes:

Decyl Glucoside - A plant-based cleanser used in skincare and baby products.

Organic Chamomile -An organic flower extract with soothing properties.

Coco-Glucoside - A very gentle cleanser derived from corn, coconut and/or palm.

Sodium Citrate - A biodegradable salt that acts as a water softener.

Sodium Bicarbonate - A mineral-based water softener also known as baking soda!

Sodium Phytate - A natural binder that prevents minerals from interfering with the formula.

To try these in your home go to:
https://thebiblicalnutritionist.com/natural-house-cleaning/

Shaklee – A company that has been in the forefront of safe cleaning products since 1960. This was before green clean was even a word. The two products Basic H2 and Basic G are safe, economical and work. They are safe around babies and even puppies. The concentrated formula is perfect for prepping since one bottle can last up to 3-4 years.

Shaklee Basic H2 This little 16 ounce bottle creates an unbelievable 48 gallons of safe, powerful all-purpose cleaner.

Germ Fighter

Almost every prepper website makes chlorine a mandatory product. Although I have chlorine on hand for emergency use my preferable product of choice is one that kills germs but yet is not toxic to breathe or can cause skin or hormone issues. Don't get me wrong, I don't want harmful bacteria in my water or around my home but there are safer and more powerful options. This is where the Shaklee Basic G is a good option. I am not affiliated with Shaklee so you can find a distributor through the internet.

Basic G – Germ Off Tough on germs! Bacteria, fungi and viruses can wreak havoc on your family's health and safety. Used as directed, Basic G tackles over 50 of those pesky microbes, including several animal viruses. That makes it a good choice for use in the kitchen, bathroom or pet area. One quart bottle makes 64 gallons. Yes, that is not a typo.

What to have on hand for cleaning

Laundry detergent - Make it or buy premade, the choice is up to you. Here are some items that would be helpful to have on hand for cleaning the home and doing laundry without power.

When cleaning with Branch Basics it is helpful to also buy the spray bottles. With the clear label of mixture and usage, even kids will be able to know which bottle to use for a specific purpose.

Cleaning cloths – the best type of cleaning cloth is the micro fiber. They can be used over and over and laundered over 400 times. They will last till the rapture.

Laundry without power—Okay, let me just say I hope this doesn't happen. But if it does then supplies will be needed.

Yes, we can use our kitchen sinks for small clothes but for larger clothes we will need a large bucket. The six gallon buckets will work for this or the old wash pan seen in old movies or at the antique store. Having two buckets will allow a wash and rinse.

To wring out the clothes I learned from one fellow prepper to use the yellow mop bucket on wheels used in restaurants with the squeeze handle at the top. That is perfect!

Clothes line. I love drying my linens outside to get the fresh breeze smell. One of my most favorite things is to climb into my bed with fresh air dried sheets. To do this I have bought from Lowes a retractable clothes line. It is simple to pull out from the corner of my screened porch and then stretch to a tree where I have a hook. Hang up the clothes or sheets, let them dry and then when they are done, I snap the clothes line back in the holder. No one who comes to my house knows I have a clothes line ready to go. Don't forget the clothes pins.

Conclusion

Pray about this cleaning information. It makes sense to start using these today since they are a healthier option.

Plan - What types of products are best for your family? What is easier – making your own or buying economical safe cleaners? Also note the amount needed for long term situations. Do inventory of current products on hand.

Put Into Action – Purchase what is necessary to keep the family clean for at least 6 months and preferably 1 year.

Practice – Start now using products that are safer for the family and easier on the budget.

Medicine/Herbal Medicine Cabinet

The ER wait time is 25 minutes. How many times do we drive by this sign? We take the Emergency Room for granted – it will always be there. But what if it wasn't or we did not have the money to go? Or better yet, what if we want to care for our family naturally? Then here are a few suggestions.

Here is a suggested list of natural items to have on hand for medical issues:

- Baking Soda – see part B
- Alcohol – isopropyl for sterilizing
- Epsom Salt – see part B
- Hydrogen Peroxide – see part B
- *Garlic – naturally grown in your garden or supplemental
- *Alfalfa – a must for all-natural healing
- *Vitamin C – a must for numerous symptoms
- *Probiotics – to counteract unpurified water or unclean food from the garden
- Activated Charcoal – may help alleviate tooth/gum, pain/infection
- These items plus the regular first aid bandages, wraps, and bandages.
- *Multi-Vitamin – every member of the family needs to be on a high quality multi vitamin

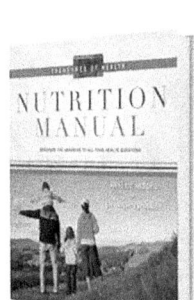

*These items are explained in great detail in the *Treasures of Health Nutrition Manual*.

First Aid Kits

First aid kits are **necessary** for each vehicle and for the home. Make sure they are well stocked and always replenished when used.

These kits can be purchased prepackaged or we can assemble our own. I have found the prepackaged kits to be economical and then supplemented with items I need more.

Make sure to have gloves, scissors and tape in each kit besides the usual bandages and dressing items.

Alcohol wipes, hand cleaners, stomach digestive aids and Tylenol are also essential to have in each location as well.

If a family member takes prescriptions, a list of all prescriptions in each kit will be very handy.

Build an Herbal Medicine Library

> *And he showed me a [a]pure river of water of life, clear as crystal, proceeding from the throne of God and of the Lamb.² In the middle of its street, and on either side of the river, was the tree of life, which bore twelve fruits, each tree yielding its fruit every month. The leaves of the tree were for the healing of the nations.*
> *Revelation 22:1-2 (NKJV)*

The leaves were for the healing. From the beginning of creation till the last chapter in the Bible we see herbal remedies mentioned for healing. Herbs include: flowers, stems, berries, and roots of plants to prevent, relieve, and treat illness.

There are more than 750,000 plants on earth. Very few have been studied scientifically. With plants being God's design it is helpful to consider the power of a plan lies in the interaction of all its ingredients. Plants used as medicines offer synergistic interactions between ingredients both known and unknown.

Before the pharmaceutical revolution in the early 1900's plants were considered the healing element everyone from grandma to the doctor understood.

Yet today, even to mention an herb for healing is considered unconventional or unscientific. The family who is educated in herbs is the family that will fare well in the coming days.

Here is a list of suggested books to gather in your library now and begin to grow and learn.

Holistic Herbal; A Safe and Practical Guide to Making and Using Herbal Remedies by David Hoffman

This book teaches how to make herbal remedies with plants we may grow and harvest.

Smart Medicine for a Healthier Child by Janet Land

Smart Medicine shares safe and effective relief of common childhood disorders, using natural supplements, herbs, homeopathy, and diet. If you have children in your life then this book should be on your shelf.

Treasures of Health Nutrition Manual by Annette Reeder and Dr Richard Couey.

How to Raise a Healthy Child in Spite of Your Doctor by Dr. Mendelsohn

Digestive Wellness 5th edition By Elizabeth Lipski

Conclusion

Pray about the topic of Herbal Medicine and how you can start using this information today.

Plan - Learn about herbs and their nutritional benefits.

Put Into Action – Take inventory of products already in the medicine cabinet. Purchase what is needed. Remember everyone needs to be taking a high quality multi vitamin. Most prepper websites refer to products that are filled with preservatives and additives. This will not contribute to health during a crisis but create more dis-harmony in the body. Choose wisely.

Practice - Practice making a garlic or onion warm liquid. This remedy has helped numerous people and children are relieved of infection.

Dan Celia Comments

From the Dan Celia website.

Remember, it is better to be prepared for the worst and pray for the best...

- **FOOD** - During a catastrophe, they say it will take approximately *three hours* for grocery stores to be void of all food, and approximately *three weeks* to recover that. Have an absolute **minimum of two months' worth of food** in case catastrophe hits.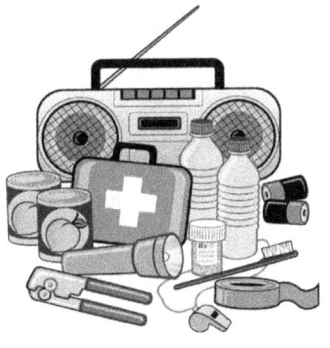
- **GASOLINE** - There will be panic in the streets - chaos. Be prepared to stay indoors and have food, water and enough *gasoline* to get you where you may have to go in an emergency.
- **MONEY** - Have *cash* on hand *in the home*. Have some cash available since cash may be hard to get a hold of and this may be your best chance of bartering. Consider having some *foreign currency* on hand. As the dollar devalues, some foreign currency (like the Swiss Franc) may hold its value and be able to buy more goods than the dollar will.
- **HEAT** - Remember, in a catastrophe we could *lose electricity* or, if nothing else, be experiencing rolling blackouts. If it is at a time during the cold weather, you must be prepared to winterize your plumbing and to have some source of heat.

- **EMERGENCY RADIO** - Have an *Emergency Radio* - preferably one that gets its energy from a crank on the side or solar power - since that may be our only communication with the outside world for a period of time. Also, have an antenna for your television. You can buy them at Best Buy, Wal-Mart and other places. A simple antenna that plugs into most televisions may be another source of communication if there is electricity.
- **MEDICINE**- Some of you have medical needs for certain medicines that you need to take every day. You must make sure that you have an adequate supply of medicines. Some prescription drugs that you use daily can be filled in three or six month supplies. I would check with your doctor to see if that is a possibility. Also, check the expiration date on the medicines that you have.
- **FIRST AID** - Make sure that you have *first aid* supplies, such as antibiotic ointments, bandages, Tylenol and other over-the-counter medications.
- **GENERATOR** - It would be ideal to be able to have even a *small portable generator* - preferably one that, again, runs off solar power. This would eliminate the need for fuel. Remember, if you have a generator that uses gasoline or propane, use it sparingly - only for emergencies and only when absolutely necessary. We will have no way of knowing whether it will have to last two months or a year, so always assume that it is going to be for a very long period of time.
- **GUN** - I happen to be a believer that everyone should have at least one *gun* - not necessarily for protection but, again, in being prepared for an extended period of time. You would be surprised what you will learn if you need to feed your family. Remember to also have *adequate ammunition*.
- **SEEDS** - vegetable *seeds* for things that will grow in your area of the country. It may be important to be able to cultivate a small piece of ground to be able grow some of you own food supplies.
- **BARTERING** – Your food may be needed for bartering for other services since many people will not have planned ahead.

- **EXTENDED FAMILY** – If times get tough there may be more family moving in. So prepare for extras.

Consider These Two Things

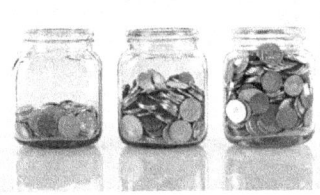

I *desperately* urge you to consider two things as we get deeper into 2015. **First** is *savings*. Your family's major focus should be on *savings*. Savings is *not* investing. Savings is *liquid*. Savings is in a bank or in a safe, or maybe at home in a cookie jar. But you must have *significant savings*.

Second, you need to get out of debt and stay out of debt. Do this as quickly as you can.

Building savings and becoming debt free will help you survive the ongoing *volatility* - and even worse things that may come.

Bottom Line:
- Store food.
- Store water.
- Keep some cash at home, maybe some of it in small amounts of gold or silver, Swiss Francs, Euros, or other foreign currencies that could help when things come tumbling down.

I am not talking about prepping for five years. I am talking about having enough to keep you out of the *chaos* that could ensue from an extreme economic event.

Prepare for Economic Armageddon

What if we experience more than an event? What if we experience a complete economic meltdown around the globe? An economic Armageddon. How do we prepare financially for that?

We can't, so let's not even try.

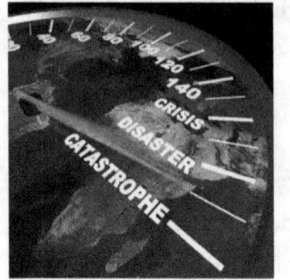

In that case, your finances - savings and everything else - will be devastated.

We can't prepare *financially* for an economic Armageddon, but we can prepare in more important ways. Mentally. Emotionally. Spiritually.

We need to be in a survival mode for our families. We need to accept what God brings and remember that He, not our finances, is our source. In an economic catastrophe, everyone will face the loss of money and possessions. As Christians, we will need to be the stable force in society. To put our faith in God . . . and help others do the same.

I know this all sounds incredibly doomsday-like, but I am concerned about this year and how it will end. Oh, I may add some things to my buy list. I may continue to talk about the markets and where they are headed . . . and you certainly need to continue to listen. I will do my best to be a *watchman* and a *warning sound* as long as the Lord allows me to do so. But . . . we must place our trust in the Lord and *not* in our savings and investments. *IF* we have an Economic Armageddon, it will not last six months or twelve months or two years. It will be *global* in nature and will last many, many years.

> As Christians, we will need to be the stable force in society. To put our faith in God... and help others do the same.

But never forget - our *true hope* lies in our Lord and Savior *Jesus Christ*. The treasures we *need* to protect and guard are the treasures we are storing in heaven. We can place our hope and find peace in that, and only in that.

Dan Celia Comments

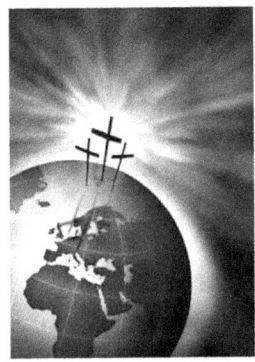

"Do not lay up for yourselves treasures on earth, where moth and rust destroy and where thieves break in and steal; **20** *but lay up for yourselves treasures in heaven, where neither moth nor rust destroys and where thieves do not break in and steal.* **21** *For where your treasure is, there your heart will be also.* (Words of Jesus in Matthew 6:19-21 NKJV)

http://www.financialissues.org/news.cfm?id=194

Praising

Praise the Lord!
Sing to the Lord a new song,
And His praise in the congregation
of the godly ones. Psalm 149:1

Our hope will always be in the Lord. Recently I was dealing with the loss of my 16 year old best friend, Millie. She was my constant companion and I had never known a dog could own such a large part of your heart. Besides losing her, my husband's employer announced they wanted 900 people to retire and vacate within 3 months. Then on top of that my family was going through a difficult upheaval. Losing my favorite pet, our income and our stability all in one short time frame caused many sleepless nights and streams of tears. This was all happening while America was turning its back on Israel and promising its pledge to Planned Parenthood's selling of baby parts.

Finally when I had voluntarily turned each of these situations over to God and TRULY trusted Him my attitude changed, my outlook changed and my praises increased. Through everything we can give praises.

I always remember the story of Corrie Ten Boom. Her sister prayed for fleas in their overcrowded concentration bunk house. When questioned why she would pray so absurdity she shared how the guards don't come in the houses with fleas. It gave them the uninterrupted time for praise and Bible study.

So praise Him during difficulties, during fleas, and during times of rejoicing. He knows all and our cells respond to the praises.

Amazing Grace

Amazing grace how sweet the sound
That saved a wretch like me
I once was lost but now am found
Was blind but now I see

The Lord has promised good to me
His Word my hope secures
He will my shield and portion be
As long as life endures

When we've been there ten thousand years
Bright shining as the sun
We've no less days to sing God's praise
Than when we'd first begun

We Are A Moment

We are a moment You are forever
Lord of the ages God before time
We are a vapor You are eternal
Love everlasting reigning on high

(CHORUS)

Holy Holy Lord God Almighty
Worthy is the Lamb Who was slain

Highest praises honor and glory
Be unto Your name
Be unto Your name

We are the broken You are the healer
Jesus Redeemer mighty to save
You are the love song we'll sing forever
Bowing before You blessing Your name

(CHORUS)

Days of Elijah

These are the days of Elijah
Declaring the Word of the Lord
And these are the days
Of Your servant Moses
Righteousness being restored
And though these are days
Of great trials
Of famine and darkness and sword
Still we are the voice
In the desert crying
Prepare ye the way of the Lord

(CHORUS)
Behold He comes
Riding on the clouds
Shining like the sun
At the trumpet call
So lift your voice

It's the year of Jubilee
And out of Zion's hill
Salvation comes

And these are the days of Ezekiel
The dry bones becoming as flesh
And these are the days
Of Your servant David

Rebuilding a temple of praise
And these are the days of the harvest
The fields are as white in the world
And we are the laborers
In Your vineyard
Declaring the Word of the Lord

(CHORUS X2)

Jesus Loves Me

Jesus loves me this I know
For the Bible tells me so
Little ones to Him belong
They are weak but He is strong

Yes Jesus loves me
Yes Jesus loves me
Yes Jesus loves me
The Bible tells me so

Jesus loves the children dear
Children far away or near
They are safe when in His care
Every day and everywhere

Yes Jesus loves me
Yes Jesus loves me
Yes Jesus loves me
The Bible tells me so

People Need the Lord x2

People need the Lord
People need the Lord
At the end of broken dreams
He's the open door

People need the Lord
People need the Lord
When will we realize
People need the Lord

Jesus Loves the Little Children

Jesus loves the little children
All the children of the world
Red and yellow black and white
They are precious in His sight
Jesus loves the little children of the world

Jesus died for all the children
All the children of the world
Red and yellow black and white
All are precious in His sight
Jesus died for all the children of the world

Praise Him Praise Him

Praise Him, praise Him
All ye little children
God is love, God is love
Praise Him, praise Him
All ye little children
God is love, God is love

Love Him, love Him
All ye little children
God is love, God is love
Love Him, love Him
All ye little children
God is love, God is love

Thank Him, thank Him
All ye little children
God is love, God is love
Thank Him, thank Him
All ye little children
God is love, God is love

To God be the Glory

To God be the glory great things He hath done
So loved He the world that He gave us His Son
Who yielded His life an atonement for sin
And opened the life gate that all may go in

Praise the Lord praise the Lord
Let the earth hear His voice
Praise the Lord praise the Lord
Let the people rejoice
O come to the Father through Jesus the Son
And give Him the glory great things He hath done

Because He Lives

God sent His Son they called Him Jesus
He came to love heal and forgive
He bled and died to buy my pardon
An empty grave is there to prove
My Savior lives

Because He lives I can face tomorrow
Because He lives all fear is gone
Because I know He holds the future
And life is worth the living
Just because He lives

How sweet to hold a newborn baby

And feel the pride and joy he gives
But greater still the calm assurance
This child can face uncertain days
Because He lives

Because He lives I can face tomorrow
Because He lives all fear is gone
Because I know He holds the future
And life is worth the living
Just because He lives

> A woman who fears
> the Lord will be praised.

How Great Is Our God w/ How Great Thou Art

How great is our God
Sing with me
How great is our God
And all will see how great
How great is our God

How great is our God
Sing with me
How great is our God
And all will see how great
How great is our God

Then sings my soul
My Savior God to Thee
How great Thou art

How great Thou art
Then sings my soul
My Savior God to Thee
How great Thou art
How great Thou art

How great is our God
Sing with me
How great is our God
And all will see how great
How great is our God!

Worshipping

I Spied God Today

The joy of the Lord will always be our strength. Even during difficult times God is still on the throne and we can be joyful. We need to be joyful for ourselves but even more importantly for our kids.

One way to do that is to play the game: I Spied God Today.

Each day ask the children how they saw God today.

Here is an example. I was driving to Washington DC today and on the radio they shared a true story of a lady in Texas who was driving along during a torrential downpour of rain. Her car was quickly caught up in a flooded situation. It began to start rocking and floating. She was stuck in the car with the windows up. Everyone around her tried to help by attempting to break open the windows and get her out. And just as it seemed no use, one man reached in through the window and grabbed her hand just before her head was almost under water and he pulled her out.

After the storm subsided and they pulled her car out of the water they were amazed at what they saw. All the windows were totally closed. None of them were open.

It was a miracle.

Now listening to that story made my heart appreciate what God is doing in lives all around us. It was a chance where I spied God working in that situation.

So I can share that story and say I spied God saving that woman's life.

Another example is when we see animals caring for their young or plants growing and producing a harvest. " I spied God when the mother bird fed her babies." " I spied God when he made the cucumber grow on the vine."

Or it could be personal "I spied God when I told the truth today." " I spied God when that young boy picked up the book a lady dropped."

" I spied God when the person accepted Jesus today."

" I spied God ……."

Ask family members "How did you see God working today?" Share that with everyone.

Together we can bring joy and blessings to each other by sharing how we see God at work. The more we focus on what He is doing the less we will be concerned with the 'me' in our situation.

An Amen Day

Today is going to be an Amen Day
I heartily agree with whatever God brings my way!

Each morning we wake up is a day we can praise the Lord. Our day can be determined by how we set our minds. For me, I wake up and say:

"Today is going to be an amen day, I heartily agree with whatever God brings my way!"

This does not mean my day will be perfect in my eyes but it does mean that nothing will happen to me that God is not already aware and working through. It is up to me to praise Him through all things.

Journal each day to help "see" how God is working. When stress happens it is easy to forget His workings in our life.

Bible Verses

If we don't have a notebook or spiral notecard collection of favorite Bible verses now would be a good time to write one. Or perhaps write out three sets of verses and place one in each back pack. Having these handy will help us be focused and prayerful.

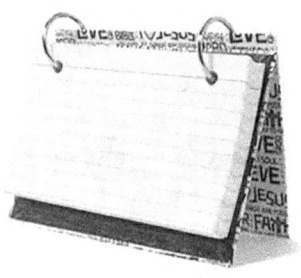

Psalm 148

Praise [b]the Lord!
Praise the Lord from the heavens;
Praise Him in the heights!
² Praise Him, all His angels;
Praise Him, all His hosts!
³ Praise Him, sun and moon;
Praise Him, all stars of light!
⁴ Praise Him, [c]highest heavens,
And the waters that are above the heavens!
⁵ Let them praise the name of the Lord,
For He commanded and they were created.
⁶ He has also established them forever and ever;
He has made a decree which will not pass away.

⁷ Praise the Lord from the earth,
Sea monsters and all deeps;
⁸ Fire and hail, snow and clouds;
Stormy wind, fulfilling His word;
⁹ Mountains and all hills;
Fruit trees and all cedars;
¹⁰ Beasts and all cattle;
Creeping things and winged fowl;
¹¹ Kings of the earth and all peoples;
Princes and all judges of the earth;

¹² Both young men and virgins;
Old men and children.

¹³ Let them praise the name of the Lord,
For His name alone is exalted;
His glory is above earth and heaven.
¹⁴ And He has lifted up a horn for His people,
Praise for all His godly ones;
Even for the sons of Israel, a people near to Him.
[d]Praise [e]the Lord!

Partnering

{ She extends her hands to the poor. }

Garden clubs seem to be a thing of the past. Let me encourage you to reinvigorate the idea. It is time to join or start a garden club of your own. Getting together with like-minded believers to share garden, cooking, and preparing tips will greatly increase your learning and fun.

It will allow chances to share appliances, the harvest and the outcome.

My spaghetti squash grew abundantly this year, so much so that I have started swapping them for foods I don't have. Our Proverbs 31 Prepper Facebook page is a great place to share your ideas and swap goods.

Networking with your garden club will let the expert lettuce grower share their crop with the orchard expert.

Sharing and swapping make prepping rewarding.

Meeting together now at least twice a month would be a good time for sharing Scriptures and stories of how God is working.

Garden clubs – or titled something you prefer is a chance to work together as teams. Share your talents; barter with each other, but most of all support each other.

Part B

Dehydration Tips

Preparing Food

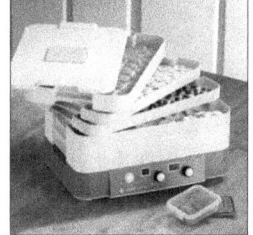

1. Try to slice or cut food all the same size so it will dry at approximately the same time. Make thin, flat cuts.
2. Don't slice food too thin. ¼-½" thickness is perfect.
3. The larger the cut area, the faster and better the food dehydrates since moisture escapes best from a cut or broken surface.
4. Thin stalked vegetables like green beans, asparagus or rhubarb should be cut in half the long way or with an extreme diagonal cut. Fruit should be sliced across the core. Place these cut side up on the tray.
5. Small fruits like strawberries can be cut in half, while even smaller berries should either be cut in half or blanched slightly to break the skin.
6. Waxy skinned fruits (i.e. – cherries, grapes, plums and blueberries must have their skins poked or pitted and will take 1-2 days to dehydrate depending on their size.
7. The peel of fruits and vegetables contain much of the nutritional value. It is better not to peel, if the dried food is to be eaten as a snack. If you are using apples in a pie or tomatoes for soup you will want to peel before dehydrating.

8. Once food has been cut or sliced fill the drying trays by arranging slices in a single layer with a little space between slices. Some tray holes must always be left uncovered for good air circulation.
9. Some foods vegetables, like beans, corn, peas and broccoli must be steam blanched before drying. Steam blanching may take from 30 – 90 seconds.
10. Fruits that turn brown when exposed to air, (apples, peaches, bananas or pears) can be dipped in solutions of orange, pineapple or lemon juice or ascorbic acid or approximately two minutes prior to drying. Drain on paper towel before placing on tray.

Filling Trays

1. Food shrinkage during dehydration may cause smaller foods to fall through holes in the drying trays. To prevent this from happening, line trays with mesh inserts.
2. To dry chopped or shredded foods, spread on mesh inserts. Food should not be spread thicker than 3/8 inch. Use a fork to expose the mesh insert in several places to provide proper air circulation.
3. Some foods such as very ripe tomatoes, citrus or sugared fruits may drip. After placing food on drying trays tap tray firmly on a towel to remove excess moisture. To catch remaining overflow, use fruit leather sheets on the bottom two trays. Alternate sheets on one half or each of the bottom trays When the food stops dripping, remove the fruit leather sheets from the bottom two trays.
4. Do not cover the center hole in the lid or trays.
5. Chili, stews, casseroles, etc. may be dried on fruit leather sheets an stored up to 3 months.

Dehydration Process

1. There is not a set time limit for drying foods. It depends on the type of food, how thick it is sliced, and the amount of water in the food.
2. When food is dried the flavors and sugars concentrate so the dried food has a much stronger flavor than fresh.

3. When using more than 4 trays periodic rotation will give optimum results.
4. Do not add seasonings or spices to vegetables until they are reconstituted and cooked.

Storing Dried Foods
1. Allow dehydrated food to cool thoroughly.
2. Dried food should be stored in a cool dry, dark place.
3. Use clean, air-tight and moisture-proof containers. Do not use cloth bags, lightweight plastic bags, bread wrappers or any container without an air-tight fitting lid. Heavy, zippered plastics bags or heat sealed bags are excellent.
4. Dried fruits and vegetables should not be stored longer than one year. Dried meats, fish, poultry or jerky should be used within a month or two.
5. Many vegetables may be powdered. Tomatoes powdered and added to water make great tomato sauce for pizzas, etc.

Reconstitution
1. To reconstitute most foods soak in water 15 minutes to 2 hours depending on the size, and use. Foods that take longest to dehydrate will take the longest to reconstitute.
2. Liquid from reconstituting food has great nutritional value. Use in soups, leathers, pies, etc.
3. To reconstitute chili or stew add hot water and let sit 15 minutes.

Temperature Tips
There are no absolutes and quite a few variables in food dehydration. The only way to become proficient is to dry, dry, and dry some more. Certain varieties of produce and humidity in the air make a difference in the drying time and quality of dried products.

Experiment with different drying temperatures, thicknesses of produce, and pre-treatment versus no pre-treatment.

Generally fruits should be dried at 130° to 140°, (135° works well). Vegetables should generally be dried at 125°. By drying foods in this temperature range you will minimize the loss of heat-sensitive vitamins A and C.

For jerky start on high (up to 160°) and half way through turn it to 140°.

Nuts and seeds are high in oil. If higher temperatures are used, they will tend to become rancid, developing off flavors. The best drying temperature for them is between 90° to 100°.

Herbs and spices are most flavorful when they first open and should be harvested while very fresh. Because the aromatic oils are very sensitive temperatures should be between 90° to 100°. Herbs generally dry in a few hours. Do not load the trays too heavily or drying time will be prolonged. Flowers should also de dried at the same temperature range to help maintain aroma and colors.

Use these guidelines for the foundation of your dehydrating techniques. Expand on them as you gain skill and confidence with the experience.

LeQuip Filter Pro Dehydrator
https://designedhealthyliving.com/shop

Market leader in dehydration technology. Unique air filtration system. Stackable to 12 trays high. This durable unit has a "solid state" variable temperature control to ensure food dries uniformly and consistently. Digital displays make it easy to read and easy to use.

Includes
- 6 Trays: 2 deep/ 4 regular
- "Clean air flow" Filter
- 6 Mesh Screens
- 2 Fruit Leather Trays
- 4 Yogurt Cups
- Instruction Book with recipes

Features
- "Clean Air" Filtration System
- 530 Watts
- Solid State Variable Temperature Control
- Micro-processor Controlled Heat Sensor (95F to 158F)
- Digital LED time and temperature Display
- Range: 95 to 158 Degrees F
- 24 Hour, Auto Shut Off timer
- 1.2 sq. feet drying space per tray. Stacks to 12 trays
- Easy to clean and use
- BPA Free
- ETL Listed

Health Benefits

Drying fruits, vegetables, jerky, and spices at home is economical and allows you to enjoy healthy snacks year round. Foods are dried without preservatives, and have concentrated flavors. Foods purchased in peak season can be dried and stored for full vitamin intake. Kids love the nutrition from fun snacks like fruit or yogurt roll-ups.

This can be purchased on the Designed Healthy Living at http://designed-healthyliving.com/shop.

Benefits of Apple Cider Vinegar

This is a short list of all the Apple Cider Uses. To get a complete list I suggest buying the book: *Apple Cider Vinegar* by Paul and Patricia Bragg.

Source: http://www.rd.com/slideshows/apple-cider-vinegar-benefits/print-view/

Apple cider vinegar benefits are plentiful. Its wide-ranging uses (rivaling the number of uses of tea tree oil and other nifty natural helpers) include everything from curing hiccups to alleviating cold symptoms, and some people have turned to apple cider vinegar to help fight diabetes, cancer, heart problems, high cholesterol, and weight issues. Read on for more reasons to keep apple cider vinegar handy in your pantry.

Helps tummy troubles.
Sip some apple cider vinegar mixed with water. If a bacterial infection is at the root of your diarrhea, apple cider vinegar could help contain the problem, thanks to its antibiotic properties. What's more, some folk remedy experts contend that apple cider vinegar contains pectin, which can help soothe intestinal spasms. Try mixing one or two tablespoons into water, or clear juice like apple juice.

Cures hiccups.
Take a teaspoonful of apple cider vinegar; its sour taste could stop a hiccup in its tracks. One teen took the hiccup remedy further and created a lollipop that includes apple cider vinegar, which she says "cancels out the message to hiccup" by overstimulating the nerves in the throat responsible for the spasms.

Soothes a sore throat.
As soon as you feel the prickle of a sore throat, employ germ-busting apple cider vinegar to help head off the infection at the pass. Turns out, most germs can't survive in the acidic environment vinegar creates. Just mix ¼ cup apple cider vinegar with ¼ cup warm water and gargle every hour or so.

Could lower cholesterol.
More research is needed to definitively link apple cider vinegar and its capability to lower cholesterol in humans, but one 2006 study found that the acetic acid in the vinegar lowered bad cholesterol in rats. Also, a Japanese study found that half an ounce of apple cider vinegar a day lowered cholesterol in people who participated in the panel.

Prevents indigestion.
Sip before eating, especially if you know you're going to indulge in foods that will make you sorry later. Try this folk remedy: add 1 teaspoon of honey and 1 teaspoon apple cider vinegar to a glass of warm water and drink it 30 minutes before you dine.

Clears a stuffy nose.
Next time you're stuffed up, grab the apple cider vinegar. It contains potassium, which thins mucus; and the acetic acid in it prevents bacteria growth, which could contribute to nasal congestion. Mix a teaspoon of apple cider vinegar in a glass of water and drink to help sinus drainage.

Aids in weight loss.
Apple cider vinegar can help you lose weight. Here's why: The acetic acid suppresses your appetite, increases your metabolism, and reduces water retention. Scientists also theorize that apple cider vinegar interferes with the body's digestion of starch, which means fewer calories enter the bloodstream.

Gets rid of dandruff.
On his website, Dr. Mehmet Oz recommends apple cider vinegar as a dandruff treatment. The acidity of apple cider vinegar changes the pH of your scalp, making it harder for yeast to grow. Mix ¼ cup apple cider vinegar with ¼ cup water in a spray bottle, and spritz on your scalp. Wrap your head in a towel and let sit for 15 minutes to an hour, then wash your hair as usual. Do this twice a week for best results.

Clears acne.
Apple cider vinegar makes a great natural toner that can leave skin looking healthier. Its antibacterial properties help keep acne under control, and the malic and lactic acids found in apple cider vinegar soften and exfoliate skin, reduce red spots, and balance the pH of your skin.

Boosts energy.
Exercise and sometimes extreme stress cause lactic acid to build up in the body, causing fatigue. Interestingly, the amino acids contained in apple cider vinegar act as an antidote. What's more, apple cider vinegar contains potassium and enzymes that may relieve that tired feeling. Next time you're beat, add a tablespoon or two of apple cider vinegar to a glass of chilled vegetable drink or to a glass of water.

Cuts down on nighttime leg cramps.
Leg cramps can often be a sign that you're low in potassium. Since apple cider vinegar is high in it, one home remedy suggests mixing 2 tablespoons apple cider vinegar and one teaspoon honey to a glass of warm water and drink to relieve nighttime leg cramps. Of course, by the time you walk to the kitchen to put the drink together, your cramp is likely to be history—but maybe that's the point.

Banishes bad breath.
If proper brushing and mouthwash doesn't do the trick, try the home remedy of using apple cider vinegar to control bad breath. Gargle with it, or drink a teaspoon (diluted with water if you prefer) to kill odor-causing bacteria.

Whitens teeth.
Gargle with apple cider vinegar in the morning. The vinegar helps remove stains, whiten teeth, and kill bacteria in your mouth and gums. Brush as usual after you gargle. You can also brush your teeth with baking soda once a week to help remove stains and whiten your teeth; use it just as you would toothpaste. You can also use salt as an alternative toothpaste. If your gums start to feel raw, switch to brushing with salt every other day.

Fades bruises.
Apple cider vinegar has anti-inflammatory properties; dabbing or laying an apple cider vinegar compress on a bruise can help fade the discoloration.

Helps control blood sugar.
A few swigs of apple cider vinegar could help keep your blood sugar levels balanced, according to several studies that have shown a link between the two. One study of people with type 2 diabetes who weren't taking insulin found that taking two tablespoons of apple cider vinegar before bed resulted in lower glucose levels by morning. Another study at the Arizona State University found that insulin resistant people who drank a mixture of apple cider vinegar and water before eating a high carbohydrate meal had lower blood sugar afterward. Scientists think the antiglycemic effect of the acid is the key.

Epsom Salt Uses

Epsom salt uses: HEALTH

This information was pulled from several books and websites.

Athlete's Foot - Soak feet in an Epsom salt bath to help relieve the symptoms of Athlete's Foot.

Remove splinters - Soak affected skin area in an Epsom salt bath to draw out the splinter.

Treat toenail fungus - Soak your affected toes in hot water mixed with a handful of Epsom salt three times a day.

Soothe sprains and bruises - Add 2 cups Epsom salt to a warm bath and soak to reduce the pain and swelling of sprains and bruises.

Ease discomfort of Gout - Ease the discomfort of gout and reduce inflammation by adding 2-3 teaspoons of Epsom salts into a basin and immersing the affected foot/joint. The water should be as hot as it is comfortable. Soak for about 30 minutes.

Detox bath: For a detoxifying bath, at least once weekly add two cups of Epsom salt to the water in a bathtub and soak for 10 minutes.

Muscle Aches & Foot odor: Mix a thick paste of Epsom salt with hot water and apply to get soothing comfort. Try soaking your aching, tired (and smelly) feet in a tub of water with half a cup of Epsom salt. Epsom salt softens skin and will even neutralize foot odor.

Epsom salt uses: BEAUTY

Exfoliate dead skin - In the shower or bath, mix a handful of Epsom salt with a tablespoon of bath or olive oil and rub all over your wet skin to exfoliate and soften. Rinse thoroughly.

Exfoliating face cleanser - To clean your face and exfoliate skin at the same time, mix a half-teaspoon of Epsom salt with your regular cleansing cream. Gently massage into skin and rinse with cold water.

Dislodge blackheads - Add a teaspoon of Epsom salt and 3 drops iodine into a half cup of boiling water. Apply this mixture to the blackheads with a cotton ball.

Remove foot odor - Mix a half cup of Epsom salt in warm water and soak your feet for 10 minutes to remove bad odor, sooth achy feet, and soften rough skin.

Remove hairspray - Combine 1 gallon of water, 1 cup of lemon juice, and 1 cup Epsom salt. Cover the mixture and let set for 24 hours. The next day, pour the mixture into your dry hair and leave on for 20 minutes before shampooing as normal.

Hair volumizer - Combine equal parts deep conditioner and Epsom salt and warm in a pan. Work the warm mixture through your hair and leave on for 20 minutes. Rinse thoroughly.

Stress Reliever Bath – Epsom salt baths three times weekly by adding 2 cups Epsom salt to a warm bath and soaking for at least 12 minutes. For the added benefit of moisturizing your skin, add 1/2 cup olive oil or baby oil. Do not use soap as it will interfere with the action of the salts. Try to rest for about two hours afterwards. If you have arthritic joints move them as much as possible after an Epsom salt bath to prevent congestion in the joints.

Epsom salt uses: HOUSEHOLD

Clean bathroom tiles - Mix equal parts Epsom salt and liquid dish detergent and use as a scrub on bathroom tile.

Prevent slugs - Sprinkle Epsom salt on or near interior entry points to prevent slugs.

As a hand wash - Mix Epsom salt with baby oil and keep by the sink for an effective hand wash.

Clean detergent build-up on washing machines - Fill the machine tub with hot water, add Epsom salt, and run an agitate/soak/agitate cycle to dissolve detergent build-up *(please consult your machine's instruction manual for specific instructions).*

Epsom salt uses: GARDENING

Fertilize your houseplants - Most plants need nutrients like magnesium and sulfur to stay in good health and Epsom salt makes the primary nutrients in most plant foods (nitrogen, phosphorus, potassium) more effective. Sprinkle Epsom salt once weekly to help nourish your houseplants, flowers and vegetables.

Keep your lawn green - Magnesium sulfate crystals, when added to the soil, provide vital nutrients that help prevent yellowing leaves and the loss of green color (magnesium is an essential element in the chlorophyll molecule) in plants. Add 2 tablespoons of Epsom salt to a gallon of water and sprinkle on your lawn to keep the grass healthy and green.

Insecticide spray - Use Epson salts on your lawn and in your garden to safely and naturally get rid of plant pests.

Baking Soda Uses

For specific directions visit: www.**arm**and**hammer**.com

Personal Care & Hygiene
- Refreshing Bath Soak
- Deodorant
- Brushes and Combs
- Hand Cleanser
- Mouth Freshening
- Foot Soak
- Hair Care
- Smelly Sneakers
- Plaque
- Oral Appliance Soak
- Facial & Body Exfoliator
- Antacids
- Teeth Cleaning
- Body Odor
- Spa Treatments

Bathroom
- Deodorizing Wastebasket
- Shower Curtains
- Septic Care
- Shower Grime
- Cleaning Bathroom Surfaces
- Cleaning Bathroom Floors
- Deodorizing Drains

Carpets & Floors
- Allergens
- Carpet Odors
- Cleaning Floors

General Household
- Clean Furniture
- Freshen Sheets
- Deodorize Gym Bags
- Upholstery Spills
- Freshen Ashtrays
- Recurrent Room Odors
- Deodorize Garbage Can
- Clean and Freshen Sports Gear
- Recyclables
- Allergens
- Freshen Upholstery
- Freshen and Deodorize Carpets
- Carpet Spills
- Freshen Closets

Kitchen
- Funky Fridge
- Greasy Dishes
- Dirty Microwave
- Coffee Maker
- Stinky Sink
- Clean & Deodorize Lunch Boxes
- Pots & Pans
- Fruit & Vegetable Scrub
- Silver Polish
- Plastic Containers
- Sponges
- Recipes
- Deodorizing Recyclables
- Dishes
- Tea Pots
- Cleaning Kitchen Surfaces
- Deodorizing Drains

- Deodorizing Fridges and Freezers
- Deodorizing Your Dishwasher

Laundry
- Cleaner Laundry
- Freshening Smelly, Musty Towels
- Laundry Stains

Garage
- Oil and Grease Stains
- Cleaning Cars
- Deodorizing Camper Water Tanks
- Deodorizing Cars

Hydrogen Peroxide

Hydrogen Peroxide is a peroxide and oxidizing agent with disinfectant, antiviral and anti-bacterial activities. It is most helpful and healthful in killing viruses and pathogens.

It is the perfect go to for numerous reasons and should be a mainstay in your home.

I keep a bottle in each bathroom, laundry room and even the kitchen.

As a daily go-to it can help with cleaning whites, getting rid of blood on clothes and quickening the healing of cuts.

Medical Benefits
- Ease a Sore Throat
- Soothe Dry Skin
- Clean and Disinfect Small Cuts
- Get Rid of Acne
- Get Rid of Canker Sores
- Get Rid of Bad Breath with a Peroxide Mouth Rinse
- Battle Foot Fungus
- Treat Colds
- Get Rid of Ear Infections
- Get Rid of Ear Wax
- Treat a Sinus Infection
- Treat a Toothache with Hydrogen Peroxide
- Detoxifying Bath
- Treating Yeast Infections
- Teeth Whitener
- Use as a Toothpaste
- Use as Deodorant
- Clean Contact Lenses
- Whiten Your Nails
- Cover Your Darker Roots
- Lighten Your Hair
- Disinfect Your Toothbrush

- Treatment for Gum Disease
- Soften Corns and Calluses on Your Feet

House Cleaning Uses of Hydrogen Peroxide
- Disinfecting Countertops
- Whiten Grout
- Clean Mirrors
- Clean Toilet
- Clean Bathroom Tiles
- Hydrogen Peroxide Kills Mold

Hydrogen Peroxide Uses in the Kitchen
- Clean Cutting Boards
- Add It to the Dishwasher
- Removes Stubborn Caked-On Food
- Disinfect Sponges and Dishrags
- Clean Fruits and Vegetables
- Keeping Fruits and Vegetables Fresh
- Keeping Salad Fresh
- Cleaning the Fridge
- Grow Mushrooms in the Refrigerator
- Cleaning Windows

Miscellaneous Uses of Hydrogen Peroxide
- Clean Your Rugs, Carpet and Mattress
- Clean Makeup Brushes
- Clean Child's Toys
- Use Hydrogen Peroxide in the Laundry Room
- Brighten Your Curtains and Table Cloths
- Wash Shower Curtains
- Remove Tough Stains from White Clothing
- Remove Odors from Your Clothes and Carpet
- Disinfect Kid's Lunchboxes
- Disinfect the Inside of a Cooler with Peroxide
- Sanitize Reusable Bags

- Clean the Humidifier or Dehumidifier
- Increase Plant Growth with Hydrogen Peroxide
- Kill Mites
- Eliminate Algae from Your Aquarium
- Help Transport Fish
- Treat Animal Wounds
- Induce Vomiting to Save Your Pet's Life
- Water Sanitation
- Remove Skunk Odors
- Get Rid of Weeds
- Cleaning Compost Buckets

Hydrogen Peroxide Benefits
- Safe and Natural Cleaning Compound
- Safe and Chemical-Free Stain Remover

For more detailed information go to: https://www.tipsbulletin.com/hydrogen-peroxide/

Top 64 Uses of a Bandana for Survival and Prepping

Bandanas are the best prepper item of all. The numerous uses make it the perfect go to. Bandanas can be bought with printed designs to make them a double blessing. Some designs to consider: animal scat markings, animal tracks, the compass of the sun, how to tie knots, how to cook on a campfire, plus more. There are many creative designs and teaching resources now available on bandanas. Most importantly is to use bandanas as a marking for your family or each individual.

Here are 64 top uses for Bandanas. You may come up with even more.

Cooking
1. To filter water
2. As a salad spinner
3. As a coffee filter
4. To open a stuck lid
5. Picnic cloth
6. As an apron
7. Wrap leftover pancakes, biscuits, etc.
8. As a pot holder when getting hot pots from the fire or stove

Personal Use
1. Absorb sweat off the forehead and eyes
2. As a mask in sandstorms, house fires, riots, etc.
3. Protect the back of the neck from sunburn
4. To color code your Back Pack - let every family member have their own color bandana
5. Camouflage your face
6. To wipe sweat and dirt from your face
7. To blow your nose
8. To keep the light out when trying to nap in the day time

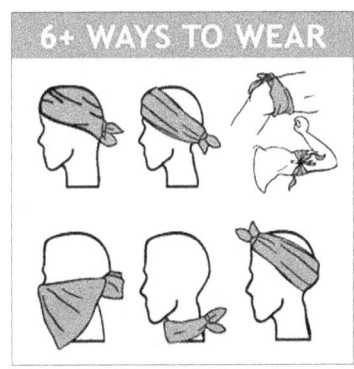

9. As a pillow – fill with leaves or soft debris and tie corners together.
10. Napkin
11. Hatband
12. To tie for a belt
13. Collect morning dew.
14. To keep your sun glasses safe
15. To wear as a disguise
16. As a toothbrush
17. Shoelaces
18. To keep hair out of your face
19. Clean your eye glasses

Medical Use

1. As a sling
2. A temporary wound dressing
3. As a tourniquet
4. As an eye patch
5. Wrap a sprained ankle or wrist
6. Tick and insect protection
7. As an insect repellant
8. To use as an ice pack

Survivor Use

1. To tie things together
2. As a cleaning cloth
3. To hold small objects by tying the corners together with tiny objects inside
4. To mark a trail
5. As a weapon – sling with rocks in it
6. As a towel
7. To get a better grip on objects
8. Kindling for starting a fire.
9. As handcuffs
10. To gag someone – ok, I hope to never need this option

11. To wave for help
12. To write stuff on
13. To check wind direction
14. Key chain
15. Replace gas cap
16. Disguise your voice over the phone
17. A drying towel for dishes
18. Hang a flashlight from tent ceiling
19. As a dog muzzle
20. As a book mark
21. As a tea bag
22. As a knife sheaf
23. To make smoke signals
24. As an 'occupied' signal outside a toilet
25. As a dog leash
26. To play tug-of-war with a dog
27. Remove oil and grease
28. As a knee pad
29. Repaid a leaky hose on the vehicle

Canning Recipes
From: *Healthy Choices*, Carlisle Press, (no author mentioned)

These recipes make a lot of quarts and pints. Have a fun cooking day with your garden club to share the products of your hands.

Cream of Mushroom Soup
1½ cup finely diced raw mushroom caps
½ Tbl. + 1 tsp. oil divided
1 cup raw mushroom caps and stems, chopped
¼ cup chopped onions
5 cups chicken stock or broth
1 cup cream
2 tsp, salt
1 Tbl. Butter
¼ tsp. garlic powder
½ cup dry milk
1½ cups water, divided
8 Tbl. Cornstarch
3 Tbl. Flour

Wash mushrooms, separate caps and stems. Finely dice raw mushroom caps and sauté in ½ Tbl. oil for 2 minutes; set aside. Coarsely chop stems and remaining caps to equal 1 cup; add chopped onions and sauté in 1 tsp. oil for 2 minutes. Put sautéed mushrooms and onions in blender, and blend until you have a smooth puree. Combine stock, remainder of cream, salt, puree, butter and garlic powder in large, heavy kettle. Combine dry milk powder with 1 cup water, stirring with whisk, and add to kettle. Heat over medium heat. Dissolve cornstarch and flour in ½ cup water. Add to hot stock mixture and stir to thicken to desired consistency. Add ½ cup sautéed mushrooms. Bring to boil and boil 5 minutes. Put in pint jars and process at 10 lb. pressure for 40 minutes.

Yield 4 pints. Can be frozen .

Canned Vegetable Soup

6-9 lbs. ground beef
- 3 quarts green and or yellow beans
- 3 quarts carrots
- 3 quarts corn
- 3 quarts peas
- 2 bunches celery
- 5 pounds potatoes
- 1 quart navy beans (soaked overnight and drained)
- 10 medium onions
- 2 medium heads cabbage
- 4 large green peppers
- 2 large red peppers
- 11 quarts tomato juice
- 1 tsp salt for each quart
- Parsley for each quart
- 1 cup pot barley, soaked overnight.

Brown ground beef until no longer pink. Dice and cook – slightly – each of the vegetables separately, then mix everything together in large container. Put soup in jar size of your choice. If vegetables seem dry when packing, add more tomato juice. Do Not overfill jars! Process 75 minutes at 10 lbs. pressure. Makes 30-35 quarts.

Enjoy this quick meal.

Resources

Books by Annette Reeder: www.TheBiblicalNutritionist.com

L'Chef Dehydrator: www.DesignedHealthyLiving.com

Notes

Proverbs 31 Prepper

Notes

Notes

Notes

Notes

Proverbs 31 Prepper

About the Author

ANNETTE REEDER ~ THE BIBLICAL NUTRITIONIST™

A uniquely qualified professional speaker and consultant, Annette is a Nutritionist and graduate of Biblical Studies. She founded Designed Healthy Living, Designed Publishing and The Biblical Nutritionist.

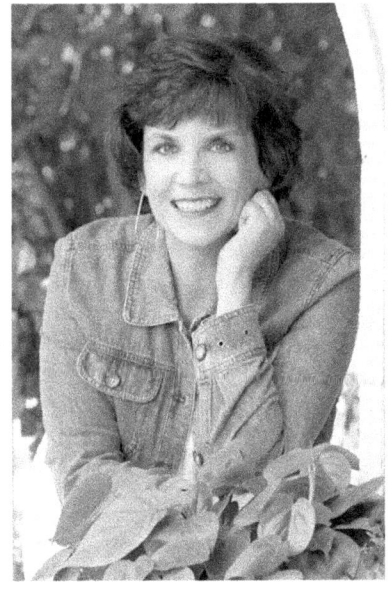

Annette's recipe starts with her creative skills from working with churches and Christian organizations, then blends them together to help each group experience flavor and fun while improving their energy and optimal health. Through her stories and lessons audiences will taste and experience how to live the life God designed - full of vitality and abundantly.

As a nutrition and health speaker from the biblical perspective, Annette shares how Scripture and nutrition intimately coincide. Each person will enjoy simple take-outs that can be applied immediately to see results.

This is a journey I have traveled for over 50 years. Join me as I share with you how to avoid the traps of counterfeit information and to experience the recipe of God's excellent health.

My journey started with the resolve that I will be forever fat! I had almost given up on being lean and healthy. Almost. But as a Christian, it was hard for me to ignore the truth – my body is the temple of the Holy Spirit and this temple was sick and fat.

With a new sense of discovery, I finally untangled myself from man's web and took a fresh look at Scripture. I was amazed at how it was completely laid out and it was the final Truth. I continue to shout Hallelujah for this Truth.

As The Biblical Nutritionist, let me lead you on this journey – no we will bypass the pits of my mistakes – and journey on toward the very pleasing reward of the Treasures of Healthy Living.

My time is spent writing, continuing studies, consulting with individuals to attain better health, and leading the amazing - life changing - Flavor of Grace Conferences.

Annette Reeder

Other Books by Annette Reeder

Treasures of Healthy Living Bible Study
By Annette Reeder and Dr. Richard Couey

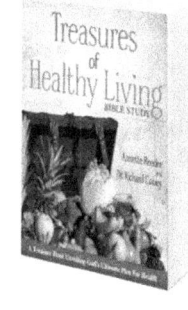

Everyone loves a treasure hunt. The hunt can be just as exciting as reaching the final treasure. This new adventure will follow the clues on our map and help us discover the answers to health to bring a life full of vitality. Watch as the counterfeits and substitutions that are currently robbing you of energy and zest are unveiled. Then what you find will fill the void with overflowing riches of health including delicious food, feelings of fulfillment, and a relationship real and personal. This Bible study will help you and your group use tools needed to reclaim health in the balance God designed.

Treasures of Health Nutrition Manual
Annette Reeder and Dr. Richard Couey

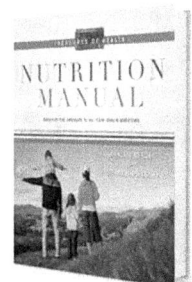

Are you tired of reading 50 books to find the answers to your health? This manual combines the nutrition from God-created foods with the value of vitamins to create a healthy and happy home and body. An encyclopedia of information is at your fingertips—a precious resource of information to treasure for years to come.

Healthy Treasures Cookbook

This cookbook brings tasty and healthy together. A collection of recipes the whole family will love.

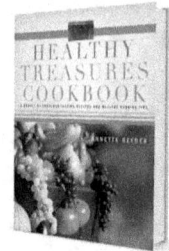

Surprise and delight will abound as you please your family with these tasty meals that will also contribute to their health and well-being. Whether you are a beginner or novice in the kitchen, this book covers it all.

Treasures of Healthy Living DVD series

The DVD series will enhance the Treasures of Healthy Living Bible study with lessons on topics such as Inflammation, Antioxidants,

Heart Health, Spiritual Health, Immune Health, Protecting Your Mind, Mindless Eating, plus creative tips on cooking with fresh herbs, making the real bread and overlooked topics such as forgiveness.

These DVDs, with over 12 hours of health living teachings, will greatly improve your understanding of God's design of your body for His kingdom.

The Daniel Fast

Fasting made simple with this complete resource with guidelines, menu plans, recipes, testimonies, journal pages and daily devotions.

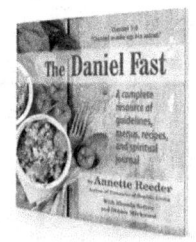

All books are available for purchase on the website: www.TheBiblicalNutritionist.com.

www.ingramcontent.com/pod-product-compliance
Lightning Source LLC
Chambersburg PA
CBHW050240120526
44590CB00016B/2165